Foreword

In a world that is constantly in motion, where the demands of daily life often overshadow the need for self-care, the importance of healthy living has never been more critical. "The Art of Wholesome Living: 10 Pillars of Vitality" is a book that arrives not a moment too soon, offering a timely, comprehensive guide to navigating the complexities of maintaining health and vitality in our modern era.

The essence of this book lies in its holistic approach to wellness. In a culture inundated with quick fixes and fleeting trends, this book stands as a beacon of balanced, sustainable living. It reminds us that health is not a destination but a continuous journey, one that encompasses the physical, mental, emotional, and social aspects of our lives.

Healthy living is often perceived as a solitary pursuit, a series of personal choices made in the quest for longevity and physical well-being. However, this book redefines that perception, presenting health as a tapestry woven from various threads that include nutrition, physical activity, mental wellness, and social connections. It acknowledges that our health is deeply intertwined with the environment we live in and the relationships we nurture.

The ten pillars outlined in this book are not just principles; they are invitations to engage with life more fully and mindfully. They encourage us to look beyond the superficial layers of health and delve into the profound impact of our daily habits and choices. Each chapter in this guide is a step towards understanding how these pillars support and strengthen each other, creating a robust structure for a fulfilling life.

One cannot overstate the significance of a balanced diet in the quest for health. Our relationship with food is complex and often fraught with misinformation and fads. This book demystifies nutrition, offering clear, actionable guidance on how to nourish our bodies with a variety of wholesome foods. It champions the idea that eating well is not about deprivation but about celebrating the abundance of nourishing options available to us.

Physical activity, another pillar, is presented not just as a means to an end but as an integral part of a joyful life. The book explores how regular exercise benefits not only the body but the mind and spirit. It underscores the idea that movement should be a joyful celebration of what our bodies can do, rather than a punitive measure for what we have eaten.

Sleep, often overlooked in our busy lives, is brought to the forefront. This book highlights the transformative power of rest, emphasizing that quality sleep is as vital to our health as diet and exercise. It provides insights into the profound ways in which adequate sleep can enhance our daily functioning and overall well-being.

Hydration, stress management, avoiding harmful habits like smoking and excessive alcohol consumption, regular health check-ups, mental health awareness, maintaining a healthy weight, and nurturing social connections are the other pillars that this book thoughtfully addresses. Each topic is explored with depth and compassion, recognizing that every individual's journey towards health is unique.

The narrative weaves these tenets together, illustrating how they collectively contribute to a vibrant, healthy life. It acknowledges the challenges and obstacles that often impede our path to wellness and offers practical, realistic strategies to overcome them. The book doesn't just impart knowledge; it inspires action. It empowers readers to take charge of their health, to make informed decisions, and to cultivate habits that enrich their lives.

As we navigate the complexities of the 21st century, where the sedentary lifestyle, processed foods, and digital overload have become the norm, this book serves as a much-needed compass. It directs us back to the basics, to the timeless principles of healthy living that can help us thrive in an ever-changing world.

The Art of Wholesome Living: 10 Pillars of Vitality is more than a manual for healthy living; it is a manifesto for a life lived with purpose, joy, and balance. It is a reminder that each day presents a new opportunity to embrace healthier choices, to connect more deeply with ourselves and others, and to appreciate the gift of health.

As you turn the pages of this book, you are embarking on a journey. It is a journey of discovery, of learning, and most importantly, of transformation. This book is your guide, your mentor, and your companion on this journey. May it inspire you to build the pillars of vitality in your own life and experience the profound joy and fulfillment that comes from living wholesomely.

Table of Contents

Foreword...1

Introduction...8

Chapter 1: A Balanced Diet 9

The Cornerstone of Health: Understanding a Balanced Diet 9

The Importance of Nutritional Diversity.................................10

Limiting Unhealthy Choices 11

Practical Tips for a Balanced Diet 12

Overcoming Challenges 15

Conclusion 15

Chapter 2: Regular Exercise 15

Embracing Movement: The Key to Physical and Mental Well-Being
....15

Understanding the Importance of Regular Exercise.....................16

The Guidelines: 150 Minutes of Moderate or 75 Minutes of Vigorous
Activity 16

The Benefits of Regular Exercise 18

Integrating Exercise into Your Lifestyle.................................20

Overcoming Barriers to Exercise 21

Conclusion 22

Chapter 3: Adequate Sleep..23

The Pillar of Rest: Unveiling the Power of Sleep 23

Understanding the Importance of Sleep..................................23

The Benefits of Adequate Sleep...25

How Much Sleep Do We Need? 27

Strategies for Achieving Quality Sleep...................................28

Overcoming Sleep Challenges 30

The Impact of Sleep Deprivation 31

Conclusion 32

Chapter 4: Hydration 32

The Role of Water in the Body 32

Understanding Dehydration 34

The Hydration Equation: How Much Water Do We Need?.............36

Hydration Strategies for Optimal Health 36

Overcoming Barriers to Adequate Hydration 38

Conclusion 40

Chapter 5: Stress Management 40

Navigating the Storms: Embracing Calm in Chaos............................40

Understanding Stress 40

The Art of Meditation 42

The Harmony of Yoga 43

Engaging in Relaxing Hobbies 45

Holistic Stress Management...47

Conclusion 49

Chapter 6: Avoid Smoking and Limit Alcohol 49

Steering Clear of Harm: A Journey Towards Healthier Habits.........49

Understanding the Impact 49

The Path to Quitting Smoking 51

Moderating Alcohol Intake 52

Building a Support System 53

Dealing with Relapse 55

Conclusion 57

Chapter 7: Regular Health Check-ups...57

The Proactive Path: Embracing Preventive Healthcare 57

Understanding Preventive Healthcare...57

The Lifesaving Potential of Screenings 58

Integrating Check-ups into Your Lifestyle................................59

Personalized Healthcare..60

The Importance of a Trusted Healthcare Provider 61

Navigating Health Anxiety 62

The Role of Lifestyle in Preventive Healthcare 62

Overcoming Barriers to Regular Check-ups 63

Health Literacy: Understanding and Advocacy 63

The Ripple Effect of Regular Check-ups 64

Conclusion 65

Chapter 8: Mental Health Awareness 66

Embracing Mental Wellness: A Journey to Inner Peace 66

Understanding Mental Health 66

Recognizing the Importance of Mental Health 67

Indicators of Mental Health Issues...68

Strategies for Maintaining Mental Well-being........................70

The Role of Professional Help 72

Overcoming Barriers to Seeking Help 75

The Impact of Lifestyle on Mental Health 76

The Importance of Self-Care...78

Conclusion 79

Chapter 9: Maintain a Healthy Weight 80

Nurturing Your Body: A Balanced Approach to Weight..................80

Understanding Healthy Weight..80

The Role of a Balanced Diet 81

Regular Exercise: A Key Component 82

The Psychology of Weight Management..................................83

Overcoming Weight Loss Challenges......................................84

The Impact of Lifestyle..85

The Role of Community and Support...87

The Health Benefits of Maintaining a Healthy Weight.....................88

Conclusion 88

Chapter 10: Social Connections...89

The Fabric of Our Lives: The Importance of Social Bonds 89

Understanding the Impact of Social Connections 89

Nurturing Family Relationships...90

The Value of Friendships...92

The Role of Community 94

Communication: The Heart of Relationships....................................95

The Digital Age and Social Connections 97

Overcoming Social Isolation..99

The Joy of Giving Back 101

Conclusion 103

Final Thoughts 103

Introduction

We embark on a journey to explore the essentials of maintaining and enhancing overall well-being. The fast-paced nature of our modern world often makes the quest for health and vitality seem daunting. Yet, the path to a fulfilling and vibrant life rests on fundamental principles that are both timeless and universally applicable.

At the heart of this book lies the understanding that a fulfilling life is built on a foundation of multiple interrelated aspects of health and wellness. We begin with the cornerstone of a balanced diet. The food we eat is more than just sustenance; it's the fuel that powers our existence. A harmonious blend of fruits, vegetables, whole grains, lean proteins, and healthy fats forms the bedrock of our physical and mental vitality. This journey through nutrition is not just about limiting processed foods and sugars; it's an invitation to embrace food as a source of nourishment, pleasure, and health.

Physical activity is the next pillar of a wholesome life. We delve into how regular exercise, whether it's moderate aerobic activity or more vigorous pursuits, is not merely a tool for maintaining a healthy weight but a catalyst for mental clarity and emotional stability. Alongside this, the importance of adequate sleep is illuminated. Quality sleep is not a luxury but a necessity, acting as the body's time for recharging, healing, and rejuvenating.

The book also highlights the critical role of hydration. Water, the essence of life, is central to everything from digestion to maintaining energy levels. We explore simple practices that keep you well-hydrated and energized. Equally important is the management of stress. Life inevitably brings stress, but it doesn't have to dominate your existence. We look at techniques like meditation, yoga, and engaging in relaxing hobbies to help you find calm amidst the chaos.

Addressing lifestyle choices, we tackle the impact of smoking and excessive alcohol consumption on health. The journey includes strategies for quitting smoking and moderating alcohol intake, leading to significant improvements in health. Alongside this, the importance of regular health check-ups is emphasized. Preventive healthcare and regular screenings are life-saving aspects of a wholesome lifestyle.

Mental health is as crucial as physical health. This guide addresses the importance of being mindful of your mental well-being and the necessity of seeking professional help when needed. In conjunction with mental health, maintaining a healthy weight is explored. This isn't about chasing an ideal but nurturing your body through a balanced diet and regular exercise.
Finally, the book underscores the importance of strong social bonds. Nurturing relationships with family and friends is not just beneficial but essential for mental health, providing support and joy in life's journey.

The Art of Wholesome Living: 10 Pillars of Vitality is more than a guide; it's a companion in your journey toward a healthier, more balanced, and joyful life. It advocates for small, sustainable changes that lead to profound transformations. Embrace these principles, and embark on a journey to discover the art of living wholesomely.

Chapter 1: A Balanced Diet

The Cornerstone of Health: Understanding a Balanced Diet

A balanced diet forms the cornerstone of good health. It is the foundation upon which our physical, mental, and emotional well-being is built. In its simplest form, a balanced diet means eating a variety of foods in the right proportions to obtain the optimal mix of nutrients that our bodies need to thrive.

This chapter delves into the essence of a balanced diet, exploring the reasons why it's crucial, what constitutes a balanced diet, and how to practically integrate it into daily life. We will unravel the complexities surrounding nutrition and provide clear, actionable insights to help you embark on a journey toward better health through mindful eating.

The Importance of Nutritional Diversity

Nutritional diversity is crucial for a healthy life. It ensures that the body receives a wide range of essential nutrients, including vitamins, minerals, and antioxidants, necessary for maintaining health and preventing diseases. A diverse diet supports optimal functioning of various body systems, from the immune system to the digestive tract. It also helps in reducing the risk of nutrient deficiencies and chronic diseases like heart disease, diabetes, and cancer.

Fruits and Vegetables

Fruits and vegetables are central to a nutritious diet. They are loaded with essential nutrients that the body needs to function optimally. The diversity in colors of fruits and vegetables is not just appealing to the eye but also represents a variety of nutrients. For instance, orange and yellow fruits and vegetables are typically high in vitamins C and A, while purple and blue options are rich in antioxidants. Integrating a mix of fruits and vegetables in the diet ensures a comprehensive intake of these nutrients. They also provide dietary fiber, which aids in digestion and maintains gut health. Regular consumption of a variety of fruits and vegetables can lower the risk of chronic diseases, support weight management, and improve overall health.

Whole Grains

Whole grains are a vital component of a healthy diet. They are rich in fiber, which aids in digestion and helps in maintaining a healthy weight. The fiber in whole grains also plays a role in lowering cholesterol levels and reducing the risk of heart disease. Whole grains provide essential B vitamins, minerals like iron and magnesium, and even some protein. Including a variety of whole grains in the diet, such as quinoa, oats, and barley, ensures a balanced intake of these nutrients and helps in maintaining energy levels throughout the day.

Lean Proteins

Proteins are essential for the growth, repair, and maintenance of body tissues. Lean proteins provide the necessary amino acids without excess calories or unhealthy fats. Animal sources like chicken, turkey, and fish are high-quality proteins, with fish also offering the benefit of heart-healthy omega-3 fatty acids. Plant-based proteins, such as beans, lentils, and tofu, not only provide protein but also fiber, vitamins, and minerals. Including a variety of protein sources ensures a balanced intake of essential amino acids and other nutrients.

Healthy Fats

Fats are essential for the absorption of fat-soluble vitamins and provide a source of energy. Unsaturated fats, particularly monounsaturated and polyunsaturated fats, are beneficial for heart health. They help in reducing bad cholesterol levels and provide essential fatty acids like omega-3 and omega-6. Sources of healthy fats include avocados, nuts, seeds, and olive oil. Incorporating these into the diet supports cardiovascular health, brain function, and overall well-being.

Limiting Unhealthy Choices

In the realm of maintaining good health, one of the most important steps is to limit the intake of processed foods, sugars, and saturated fats. The modern diet often includes a high proportion of these elements, which can be detrimental to health. Processed foods, typically high in unhealthy fats, sugars, and sodium, offer little nutritional value and are linked to various health problems. High consumption of sugar and saturated fats is associated with an increased risk of developing conditions such as obesity, heart disease, and diabetes.

Processed Foods

Processed foods are a major concern in contemporary diets. These foods are often loaded with unhealthy components like trans fats, excessive sugars, and high levels of sodium, which can adversely affect health. Regular consumption of processed foods can lead to weight gain, high blood pressure, and increased cholesterol levels, which are risk factors for heart disease and stroke. Furthermore, processed foods often lack essential nutrients like vitamins, minerals, and fiber, which are crucial for overall health.

One of the primary issues with processed foods is their ease of access and convenience, making them a common choice for quick meals. However, their low nutritional value and high caloric content can lead to poor health outcomes. Additionally, processed foods can be addictive, leading to overconsumption and associated health issues.

Sugars and Saturated Fats

The high intake of sugar, particularly added sugars found in many beverages and processed foods, is a significant health hazard. Excessive sugar consumption can lead to obesity, insulin resistance, and an increased risk of type 2 diabetes. It can also contribute to dental problems and may play a role in the development of certain types of cancer.

Saturated fats, commonly found in animal products and some processed foods, are another dietary component to be consumed in moderation. High levels of saturated fat intake are linked to increased cholesterol levels, which can lead to cardiovascular diseases. While fats are an essential part of the diet, it is important to focus on healthy fat sources, such as avocados, nuts, and olive oil, which provide essential fatty acids and other beneficial nutrients.

Practical Tips for a Balanced Diet

A balanced diet is fundamental for maintaining good health, but achieving it requires practical strategies. It's not just about choosing the right foods; it's also about planning, preparation, and understanding your body's needs. Here are some practical tips that can contribute to a healthier lifestyle.

Planning and Preparing Meals

Planning and preparing meals is a cornerstone of a healthy diet. This approach allows for more thoughtful food choices, ensuring a variety of nutrients are included in your diet. By planning meals, you can incorporate a range of fruits, vegetables, whole grains, lean proteins, and healthy fats, leading to more balanced and nutritious meals.

Meal planning also helps in controlling portion sizes and reducing food waste. It allows for more efficient grocery shopping, as you can buy exactly what you need. This not only saves time and money but also ensures that fresh and wholesome ingredients are used.

Preparing meals at home has the added advantage of control over the ingredients. This means you can avoid excessive salt, sugar, and unhealthy fats often found in restaurant meals or processed foods. Cooking methods can also be healthier, such as grilling, steaming, or baking instead of frying.

Moreover, meal planning and preparation can be a creative and enjoyable process. It encourages culinary exploration and can be a way to involve family members in healthy eating habits.

Reading Nutrition Labels

Reading nutrition labels is an essential skill for making informed food choices. These labels provide crucial information about the nutritional content of foods, including the amount of calories, fats, sugars, and sodium, as well as vitamins and minerals.

Understanding these labels can help in choosing healthier options. For instance, comparing labels can help you choose products with lower amounts of added sugars, unhealthy fats, and sodium - all of which are important for heart health and overall well-being.

Labels also provide information on the serving size, which is key for portion control. This helps in understanding how much of each nutrient you are consuming and whether it fits into a balanced diet.

Furthermore, nutrition labels can guide those with specific dietary needs, such as low sodium for blood pressure management or higher fiber for digestive health. They can also be a tool for those trying to manage conditions like diabetes, by monitoring carbohydrate intake.

Portion Control

Portion control is a vital aspect of a balanced diet. Consuming portions that are too large, even of healthy foods, can lead to weight gain and associated health problems.

Understanding serving sizes and being mindful of the amount of food you consume can help maintain a healthy weight and improve overall health. Using smaller plates, measuring servings with measuring cups, and being aware of the standard serving sizes can help in managing portions.

It's also important to listen to your body's hunger and fullness cues. Eating slowly and mindfully can help you recognize when you are full, reducing the likelihood of overeating.

Portion control doesn't mean depriving yourself; it's about eating enough to satisfy your body's needs without excess. It can also involve balancing out meals throughout the day to prevent overeating at any one meal.

Hydration

Hydration is often overlooked in discussions about a balanced diet, but it's a key component of overall health. Water is essential for nearly every bodily function, including digestion, nutrient absorption, and the elimination of waste products.

Drinking enough water can also aid in weight management. Sometimes, the body can confuse thirst with hunger, leading to overeating. Staying well-hydrated helps in differentiating hunger from thirst.

The general recommendation of eight glasses a day is a good starting point, but individual needs can vary based on factors like physical activity, climate, and overall health. Including other sources of hydration like fruits and vegetables, which have high water content, can also contribute to overall fluid intake.

Hydration is crucial for maintaining energy levels, supporting cognitive functions, and even for skin health. It's a simple yet effective component of a healthy lifestyle.

Overcoming Challenges

Adopting a balanced diet can be challenging, especially in a world filled with fast food and convenience items. However, small, gradual changes can lead to significant health improvements. Start by introducing more fruits and vegetables into your meals, switching to whole grains, and choosing healthier protein sources. Be patient with yourself and remember that making healthy choices is a lifelong journey.

Conclusion

A balanced diet is a key to a healthy life. It provides the body with the essential nutrients needed for growth, repair, and optimal functioning. By embracing a variety of fruits and vegetables, whole grains, lean proteins, and healthy fats, and limiting processed foods, sugars, and saturated fats, you can significantly improve your health and well-being. Remember, the journey towards a healthier life is a series of small steps. Each healthy choice you make is a step in the right direction.

Chapter 2: Regular Exercise

Embracing Movement: The Key to Physical and Mental Well-Being

In the journey towards optimal health, regular exercise stands as a pivotal element. It is not just about maintaining a healthy weight or building physical strength; exercise profoundly impacts our mental and emotional well-being. This chapter delves into the essence of regular exercise, understanding its importance, exploring various forms, and offering practical advice on integrating it into your daily life.

Understanding the Importance of Regular Exercise

Exercise is a powerful tool that enhances almost every aspect of health. It improves cardiovascular health, strengthens muscles, boosts mental health, and can even extend your lifespan. Regular physical activity is known to reduce the risk of chronic diseases such as heart disease, diabetes, and certain cancers. It also plays a critical role in weight management and mental health, improving mood and reducing symptoms of anxiety and depression.

The Guidelines: 150 Minutes of Moderate or 75 Minutes of Vigorous Activity

Regular physical activity is a key component of a healthy lifestyle, with established guidelines suggesting at least 150 minutes of moderate aerobic activity or 75 minutes of vigorous activity each week. Understanding and applying these guidelines can significantly contribute to overall health and well-being.

Moderate Aerobic Activity

Moderate-intensity aerobic activities are those that raise the heart rate and cause you to breathe faster while still allowing you to maintain a conversation. Examples include brisk walking, leisurely cycling, dancing, and water aerobics. These activities are particularly beneficial as they can be easily integrated into daily life, such as walking or biking to work, taking the stairs instead of the elevator, or engaging in a dance class.

Engaging in moderate aerobic activities has numerous health benefits. It improves cardiovascular health by strengthening the heart and lungs and increases endurance. It also helps in regulating blood pressure and cholesterol levels. Additionally, moderate exercise can improve mood, reduce stress, and enhance sleep quality, contributing to overall mental health.

For those new to exercise or returning after a period of inactivity, moderate activities are an excellent starting point. They are less intimidating and easier to sustain, making it more likely for individuals to stick to a regular exercise routine.

Vigorous Aerobic Activity

Vigorous-intensity activities are more challenging and require a higher level of effort. They lead to rapid breathing and a significant increase in heart rate. Examples include running, swimming laps, cycling at a fast pace, playing competitive sports, or participating in high-intensity interval training (HIIT).

These activities offer more significant health benefits in a shorter duration compared to moderate activities. They are particularly effective in improving cardiovascular fitness, building endurance, and increasing muscle mass. Vigorous exercise also has a higher calorie-burning rate, which is beneficial for weight loss and obesity prevention.

Vigorous activities are more suited to those who already have a base level of fitness and are looking to challenge themselves further. It's important to gradually increase the intensity of exercise to prevent injury and to allow the body to adapt.

Strength Training Exercises

Strength training, or resistance training, is an integral part of an exercise regimen. It involves activities that use resistance, like weight lifting, resistance bands, or body-weight exercises (like push-ups and squats), to build muscle strength and endurance.

Incorporating strength training at least twice a week has several health benefits. It helps in building and maintaining muscle mass and bone density, which is particularly important as one ages. It also enhances metabolic rate, aids in weight management, and improves body composition.

Strength training is not only beneficial for athletes but is also crucial for everyday functional fitness. It helps in performing daily tasks more efficiently and reduces the risk of injuries. Moreover, it has been shown to improve posture, balance, and stability.

The Benefits of Regular Exercise

Maintaining a Healthy Weight

Exercise is a fundamental aspect of weight management. Regular physical activity helps burn calories and fat, boosts metabolism, and increases muscle mass. Muscle tissue burns more calories than fat tissue, so increasing muscle mass through exercise aids in more efficient calorie burning, even at rest.

In addition to burning calories, regular exercise helps in regulating appetite. It can lead to improved body composition by reducing fat mass and increasing muscle mass, which is key for maintaining a healthy weight.

Exercise also has psychological benefits that contribute to weight management. It can improve mood, reduce stress, and increase self-esteem, all of which can reduce emotional eating and improve dietary choices.

Regular physical activity, when combined with a balanced diet, is the most effective way to maintain a healthy weight and prevent obesity. It's not just about the number of calories burned during exercise but also about the long-term metabolic and behavioral changes that support a healthy lifestyle.

Engaging in a combination of aerobic and strength training exercises is ideal for weight management. While aerobic exercises help in burning calories and improving cardiovascular health, strength training builds muscle mass and enhances metabolic rate. This combination ensures a balanced approach to maintaining a healthy weight.

Improving Mood and Mental Health

Regular physical activity has a profound impact on mood and mental health. Exercise stimulates the release of endorphins, serotonin, and dopamine in the brain, which are chemicals associated with feelings of happiness, relaxation, and well-being. This biochemical response can lead to a reduction in feelings of depression, anxiety, and stress.

Regular exercise also plays a significant role in improving self-esteem and self-image. As individuals exercise, they often see improvements in muscle tone, strength, and endurance, which can boost confidence and body image. Furthermore, the achievement of fitness goals, no matter how small, can provide a sense of accomplishment and increase self-esteem.

Exercise has been shown to have cognitive benefits as well. It enhances brain function, which can improve memory, attention, and problem-solving skills. Regular physical activity can also slow down the cognitive decline associated with aging and can reduce the risk of developing cognitive impairments and dementia.

For those struggling with mental health issues, exercise can be a valuable part of a treatment plan. It can serve as a complementary therapy for managing mild to moderate depression and anxiety. Additionally, the social aspects of certain types of exercise, like group sports or fitness classes, can provide social support and combat feelings of loneliness or isolation.

Reducing the Risk of Chronic Diseases

Engaging in regular physical activity is one of the most effective ways to prevent and manage chronic diseases. Exercise plays a crucial role in cardiovascular health, reducing the risk of heart disease and stroke. It helps in managing weight, lowering blood pressure, and improving cholesterol levels.

For metabolic health, regular exercise is key in preventing and managing type 2 diabetes. It improves insulin sensitivity and glucose metabolism, which helps in controlling blood sugar levels. Exercise also plays a role in reducing the risk of certain types of cancer, such as breast, colon, and lung cancer.

Musculoskeletal health is greatly improved by regular exercise. It strengthens bones, muscles, and joints, reducing the risk of osteoporosis and arthritis. It also improves balance and coordination, which is crucial in preventing falls, especially in older adults.

In terms of mental health, exercise has been shown to reduce the risk of developing depression and can improve the quality of life for those living with mental health conditions. Moreover, regular physical activity can enhance cognitive function and may reduce the risk of cognitive decline and dementia in older adults.

Integrating Exercise into Your Lifestyle

Finding Activities You Enjoy

The key to maintaining a regular exercise routine is to engage in activities that you enjoy. When exercise feels like a chore, it's much harder to stay motivated. Activities like dancing, hiking, yoga, swimming, or team sports can make exercise feel more like a fun hobby than a task.

Enjoyable activities not only increase the likelihood of consistency but also contribute to mental well-being. They can offer social interaction, a sense of accomplishment, and an outlet for stress.

Setting Realistic Goals

Setting realistic and achievable goals is essential when starting an exercise regimen. These goals can be based on frequency, duration, intensity, or types of activities. Start with small, manageable goals and gradually build up as your fitness improves. This approach helps in avoiding injury and burnout, and it fosters a sense of achievement that can motivate further progress.

Creating a Routine

Consistency is key in reaping the benefits of exercise. Establishing a routine by setting aside specific times and days for workouts can help form a habit. Having a regular schedule also makes it easier to plan around other commitments and ensures that exercise is a priority.

Mixing It Up

Variety in your exercise routine keeps it interesting and challenging. Mixing different types of workouts can prevent boredom and plateauing. It ensures that all muscle groups are worked and improves overall fitness. For example, combining cardio, strength training, and flexibility exercises provides a well-rounded fitness regimen.

Listening to Your Body

It's important to listen to your body and understand its limits. While regular exercise is beneficial, overtraining can lead to fatigue and injury. Incorporating rest days into your routine allows your body to recover and can actually enhance your fitness progress.

Overcoming Barriers to Exercise

Exercise is a crucial component of a healthy lifestyle, but various barriers can make regular physical activity challenging for many individuals. Recognizing and finding ways to overcome these barriers is key to establishing and maintaining an effective exercise routine.

Lack of Time

One of the most commonly cited barriers to regular exercise is a lack of time. Many people feel that their schedules are too busy to fit in workouts. However, exercise doesn't necessarily require large blocks of time set aside each day.

Incorporating exercise into a daily routine can be an effective way to overcome this barrier. Shorter, more frequent sessions of physical activity can be just as beneficial as longer sessions. For example, a ten-minute workout in the morning, a brisk walk during a lunch break, and another short workout in the evening can add up to a significant amount of physical activity throughout the day.

Another strategy is to integrate physical activity into other daily activities. This could include walking or biking to work instead of driving, taking the stairs instead of the elevator, or doing bodyweight exercises like squats or lunges during TV commercials. These small changes can make a big difference in overall activity levels without requiring a significant time commitment.

Lack of Motivation

Maintaining motivation for regular exercise is another common challenge. To address this, setting clear, achievable goals can be very helpful. These goals should be specific, measurable, and realistic, providing a clear target to aim for. Tracking progress towards these goals can also be motivating, whether through a fitness app, a journal, or simply noting achievements on a calendar.

Exercising with a friend or in a group setting can provide additional motivation. The social aspect of group exercise can make workouts more enjoyable, and the accountability of having a workout partner can encourage regular participation. Finding an activity that is enjoyable is also crucial for sustaining motivation over time. If you enjoy what you are doing, you are much more likely to stick with it.

Physical Limitations

For individuals with physical limitations or health concerns, exercise can seem particularly daunting. However, many types of exercise can be adapted to accommodate different abilities and conditions. Consulting with a healthcare provider or a qualified fitness professional can provide insights into what types of exercise may be suitable and safe.

It's important to focus on what you can do, rather than what you can't. For example, someone with joint problems might find low-impact exercises like swimming or cycling more comfortable. Strength training can be adapted using lighter weights or resistance bands. Even gentle forms of exercise like yoga or tai chi can offer significant health benefits.

Conclusion

Regular exercise is a vital component of a healthy lifestyle. It transcends physical health, touching every aspect of our well-being. By aiming for at least 150 minutes of moderate activity or 75 minutes of vigorous activity per week, complemented by strength training, we not only maintain a healthy weight but also enhance our mood and reduce the risk of chronic diseases. Remember, the journey to regular exercise is personal and unique to each individual.

Start where you are, use what you have, and do what you can. The path to health and vitality through exercise is not just a goal; it's a continuous, rewarding journey.

Chapter 3: Adequate Sleep

The Pillar of Rest: Unveiling the Power of Sleep

Sleep, often underrated, is a fundamental pillar of health. It's during sleep that our bodies undergo essential restorative processes, affecting every aspect of our physical and mental well-being. Understanding the importance of sleep and embracing habits that promote quality sleep can have profound health benefits.

Understanding the Importance of Sleep

Sleep is an active physiological process, crucial for our overall health and well-being. It's as important as nutrition and exercise for maintaining a healthy lifestyle. Adequate sleep is vital for numerous bodily functions, including the repair of cells, rejuvenation of the brain, and regulation of hormones.

During sleep, our bodies undergo various healing processes. It's a time when the immune system is bolstered, muscle repair occurs, and energy is restored. Sleep also plays a critical role in brain function, including memory consolidation, learning, and emotional processing. It impacts mood, cognitive abilities, and decision-making skills.

Lack of sufficient sleep has been linked to various health issues, including obesity, type 2 diabetes, cardiovascular disease, and mental health disorders like depression and anxiety. It can also impair cognitive functions, reduce focus and productivity, and increase the risk of accidents.

The Sleep Cycle

The sleep cycle consists of multiple stages, each with distinct physiological and neurological features. Understanding these stages can help appreciate the complexity and necessity of sleep.

1. **Non-Rapid Eye Movement (NREM) Sleep**: This phase is divided into three stages:
    - **Stage 1 (N1)**: The transition from wakefulness to sleep, characterized by light sleep and reduced sensory awareness.
    - **Stage 2 (N2)**: A deeper sleep stage where body temperature drops, and heart rate and breathing become regular. This stage is crucial for physical restoration.
    - **Stage 3 (N3)**: The deepest sleep stage, essential for physical healing and growth. It's during this stage that the body repairs tissues, builds bone and muscle, and strengthens the immune system.
2. **Rapid Eye Movement (REM) Sleep**: This stage is associated with vivid dreams. It's crucial for mental and emotional well-being, playing a significant role in memory consolidation, learning, and mood regulation. REM sleep stimulates regions of the brain essential for learning and memory.

Each cycle of these stages lasts about 90 minutes, and multiple cycles occur each night. The balance between REM and NREM sleep is vital for a restorative sleep experience. Disruptions in the sleep cycle, such as those caused by sleep disorders, can significantly impact health.

Good sleep hygiene involves creating an environment and routine conducive to quality sleep. This includes maintaining a regular sleep schedule, ensuring a comfortable sleeping environment (dark, quiet, and cool), limiting exposure to screens before bedtime, and avoiding caffeine and heavy meals close to bedtime.

Regular physical activity and stress management techniques like meditation can also improve sleep quality. In cases of persistent sleep issues, seeking medical advice is crucial, as untreated sleep disorders can have significant health implications.

The Benefits of Adequate Sleep

Adequate sleep is a fundamental component of good health, playing a crucial role in the proper functioning of physical, mental, and immune systems. The benefits of getting enough sleep each night are extensive, affecting nearly every aspect of our well-being.

Physical Health

The importance of sleep for physical health cannot be overstated. When we sleep, our bodies undergo a range of critical maintenance processes that are essential for recovery and rejuvenation. During the deeper stages of sleep, the body engages in tissue repair, muscle growth, and protein synthesis. This restorative function is particularly important after physical exertion, such as exercise, or recovering from injuries.

Sleep is also pivotal for heart health. It helps to regulate blood pressure and cholesterol levels, both critical factors in cardiovascular health. Regular, adequate sleep has been consistently linked to a lower risk of heart disease and stroke.

Furthermore, sleep plays a significant role in metabolic functions. It helps regulate hormones that control appetite, glucose processing, and metabolism, such as insulin. Good sleep patterns are associated with a lower risk of obesity and metabolic diseases like type 2 diabetes, as they help maintain a healthy balance of these critical hormones.

Mental Health

Sleep's impact on mental health is just as significant as its physical health benefits. One of its primary functions is to aid in the processing and consolidation of memories. This aspect is vital for learning and maintaining cognitive functions. Adequate sleep supports various brain activities, including concentration, productivity, and overall performance.

Moreover, sleep has a direct influence on mood regulation. It helps balance neurotransmitters and stress hormones like cortisol, which significantly affect our emotional state. Consistent lack of sleep has been linked to an increased risk of developing mental health disorders such as depression and anxiety.

In addition to these benefits, sleep is crucial for cognitive abilities like problem-solving and creativity. It allows the brain time to reorganize and rejuvenate, leading to improved cognitive performance and enhanced creativity.

In summary, the benefits of adequate sleep are comprehensive and touch upon almost every aspect of human health. Ensuring sufficient and quality sleep is a vital strategy for maintaining good physical and mental health, aiding in everything from cellular repair and cardiovascular health to memory consolidation, mood regulation, and cognitive functioning.

Immunity

Sleep is not just a period of rest for the body; it's a critical time for the immune system to perform essential functions. During sleep, the body engages in various processes that bolster the immune system, making it a natural immune booster.

One of the key immune functions that occur during sleep is the production of cytokines. These proteins are vital for the immune response, helping the body to fight off infections, inflammation, and stress. When we sleep, the production of certain cytokines increases, especially when we're sick or stressed, allowing the body to better combat illness and recover.

Cytokines are not the only immune cells affected by sleep. The production and activity of other immune cells, like T cells, are also influenced by sleep. Adequate sleep enhances the effectiveness of these cells, allowing for a more robust immune response.

Regular, quality sleep can make the body more resilient against various illnesses. Studies have shown that people who don't get enough sleep are more likely to get sick after being exposed to viruses, such as those that cause the common cold. Good sleep also plays a role in the body's response to vaccines, with better sleep patterns leading to a stronger immune response to vaccinations.

Stress Reduction

The relationship between sleep and stress is closely interlinked, with each significantly affecting the other. Adequate sleep plays a crucial role in managing and reducing stress.

Cortisol, known as the body's primary stress hormone, follows a daily rhythm influenced significantly by the sleep-wake cycle. Adequate sleep helps regulate cortisol levels, ensuring that they peak in the morning to promote alertness and gradually decrease throughout the day, facilitating relaxation and sleepiness in the evening.

When sleep is disrupted or inadequate, this cortisol rhythm can be thrown off balance. High cortisol levels, especially in the evening, can lead to a state of hyperarousal, making it difficult to fall asleep and contributing to a cycle of stress and sleeplessness.

Adequate sleep also contributes to better mood regulation and emotional resilience. During sleep, the brain processes emotional information, which helps in managing stress more effectively. Good sleep enhances the brain's ability to cope with stressors, both minor and major, improving overall mood and reducing the risk of stress-related disorders.

Adequate sleep is crucial for maintaining strong immunity and managing stress. By ensuring consistent and quality sleep, individuals can enhance their body's ability to fight off illnesses and are better equipped to handle the stresses of daily life. This dual benefit of sleep, impacting both physical and mental health, underscores the importance of sleep as a pillar of a healthy lifestyle.

How Much Sleep Do We Need?

The amount of sleep an individual needs can vary, but for most adults, 7-9 hours of quality sleep per night is recommended. It's important to consider not just the quantity but also the quality of sleep. Factors like uninterrupted sleep, sleep consistency, and the sleep environment play a crucial role.

Understanding personal sleep needs is important. Paying attention to how you feel after different amounts of sleep can be a good indicator. Factors like mood, energy levels, and overall health can guide you to the ideal sleep duration for your body.

Strategies for Achieving Quality Sleep

Achieving quality sleep is essential for health and well-being. A good night's sleep can improve cognitive function, mood, and physical health. Here are some effective strategies for enhancing sleep quality.

Establishing a Sleep Routine

A consistent sleep routine is crucial for regulating the body's internal clock, known as the circadian rhythm. This rhythm influences sleep-wake cycles, hormone release, and other bodily functions. Going to bed and waking up at the same time each day, including on weekends, can help stabilize this internal clock, leading to better sleep quality.

Establishing a sleep routine also involves preparing your mind and body for sleep. This can include winding down activities in the evening, such as reading or listening to calming music, which signal to the body that it's time to sleep. Avoiding stimulating activities close to bedtime, like intense exercise or work-related tasks, can also help.

Creating a Restful Environment

The environment in which you sleep has a significant impact on the quality of your rest. The ideal sleep environment is cool, dark, and quiet. A cool room temperature, around 65 degrees Fahrenheit, is generally recommended for sleep, as it helps lower the body's core temperature, a signal for sleep onset.

Darkness is important for stimulating the production of melatonin, the hormone responsible for sleep. Blackout curtains or eye shades can be helpful, especially in areas with ambient light. Similarly, a quiet environment is conducive to sleep. If noise control is challenging, consider using earplugs or a white noise machine to mask external sounds.

Mind Your Diet and Exercise

Diet and exercise play a significant role in sleep quality. Heavy meals, caffeine, and alcohol close to bedtime can disrupt sleep. A light snack before bed can be beneficial, especially if it includes foods that promote sleep, like those containing tryptophan or magnesium.

Regular exercise is beneficial for sleep, but timing matters. Engaging in physical activity earlier in the day or at least a few hours before bedtime can promote better sleep. Exercise helps reduce stress and tire the body physically, preparing it for rest.

Limit Screen Time

The blue light emitted by screens from devices such as smartphones, tablets, and computers can interfere with melatonin production. Reducing screen time in the hour before bed can help the body prepare for sleep. Consider adopting a "digital curfew" where you turn off electronic devices an hour before bedtime.

Relaxation Techniques

Incorporating relaxation techniques into your evening routine can significantly improve sleep quality. Activities like reading, taking a warm bath, practicing meditation, or gentle yoga can help relax the mind and body, making it easier to fall asleep and stay asleep.

These relaxation techniques can also be beneficial for individuals who struggle with sleep-related anxiety or insomnia. Techniques such as deep breathing, progressive muscle relaxation, or guided imagery can be particularly helpful in calming the mind and preparing the body for sleep.

Overcoming Sleep Challenges

Good quality sleep is essential for health, but many individuals face sleep challenges that can adversely affect their well-being. Understanding and addressing these challenges is crucial for maintaining overall health and quality of life.

Insomnia

Insomnia, characterized by difficulty falling asleep or staying asleep, is a common sleep disorder. It can be acute (short-term) or chronic (long-term) and can arise from various causes including stress, lifestyle habits, environmental factors, or medical conditions.

To combat insomnia, good sleep hygiene is fundamental. This includes establishing a consistent sleep routine, creating a conducive sleep environment, and avoiding stimulants like caffeine and nicotine close to bedtime. It's also important to manage stress and anxiety, as they can significantly impact sleep.

Cognitive-behavioral therapy (CBT) for insomnia is an effective treatment. It involves changing thoughts and behaviors that cause or worsen sleep problems with habits that promote sound sleep. Unlike sleeping pills, CBT addresses the underlying causes of insomnia.

In some cases, medications may be prescribed, but they are generally recommended for short-term use due to potential side effects and dependence. Consulting with a healthcare provider is crucial for determining the best course of action.

Sleep Apnea

Sleep apnea is a serious condition where breathing repeatedly stops and starts during sleep. Common signs include loud snoring, morning headaches, daytime fatigue, and waking up with a dry mouth or sore throat. It's often associated with obesity, though it can affect anyone.

If sleep apnea is suspected, it's important to see a doctor. Untreated sleep apnea can lead to serious health problems like hypertension, heart disease, and diabetes. Treatment options include lifestyle changes (like losing weight and avoiding alcohol), using a continuous positive airway pressure (CPAP) machine, or surgery in severe cases.

Restless Leg Syndrome (RLS)

Restless Leg Syndrome is a neurological disorder characterized by uncomfortable sensations in the legs and an uncontrollable urge to move them. Symptoms typically occur in the evening or during periods of inactivity. RLS can lead to difficulty falling asleep and significant sleep disruption.

Managing RLS often involves lifestyle changes, such as regular exercise, maintaining a regular sleep schedule, and avoiding substances that can worsen symptoms (like caffeine and alcohol). In some cases, medications may be prescribed to relieve symptoms.

The Impact of Sleep Deprivation

The consequences of sleep deprivation are far-reaching. It impairs cognitive functions such as memory, attention, and decision-making. Chronic sleep deprivation can increase the risk of serious health issues like obesity, diabetes, cardiovascular disease, and mental health disorders.

Lack of sleep also affects mood, leading to irritability and an increased risk of depression. It can diminish the overall quality of life, affecting relationships, work performance, and the ability to enjoy daily activities.

Understanding these risks highlights the importance of addressing sleep problems. Prioritizing sleep and seeking help for sleep disorders can significantly improve an individual's health and quality of life. It's essential not only to focus on the quantity of sleep but also on its quality. Regularly getting enough restorative sleep is a key component of a healthy lifestyle.

Conclusion

Adequate sleep is a pillar of health and vitality. It's essential for physical and mental health, boosts immunity, and plays a critical role in stress management. By prioritizing sleep and adopting strategies to improve sleep quality, you can enhance your overall well-being and quality of life. Remember, sleep is not a luxury but a fundamental component of a healthy lifestyle. Embrace it, and allow your body and mind the rest they deserve.

Chapter 4: Hydration

The Essence of Vitality: Understanding Hydration

Hydration is fundamental to life and health. Water, often described as the essence of life, is not just a substance to quench thirst but a vital nutrient that nourishes every cell and supports a myriad of bodily processes. Understanding the importance of hydration is key to maintaining health and enhancing overall well-being.

The Role of Water in the Body

Water makes up about 60% of an adult's body weight and plays a crucial role in various bodily functions. It serves as a building block for cells, a solvent for chemical reactions, a carrier for nutrients and waste products, and a temperature regulator. Proper hydration is essential for every system in the body, impacting everything from brain function to metabolic processes.

Water is essential at the cellular level, aiding in the transportation of nutrients and the removal of waste. It provides the medium necessary for biochemical reactions to occur within cells.

Through perspiration, water helps regulate body temperature, keeping it within a healthy range. This is particularly important during exercise or in hot environments.

Water acts as a lubricant in the joints, reducing friction and aiding in movement, which is crucial for preventing joint pain and injuries.

Digestive Health

Water plays an essential role in maintaining digestive health, directly influencing various aspects of the digestive process. From the breakdown of food to nutrient absorption and waste elimination, water is a critical component in the efficient functioning of the digestive system.

During digestion, water aids in breaking down food, making it easier for the body to absorb nutrients. The process of digestion begins in the mouth, where water in saliva starts breaking down food. In the stomach and intestines, water continues to facilitate the breakdown process, ensuring that nutrients are efficiently extracted from the food we eat.

Water-soluble vitamins and minerals, such as vitamin C and the B vitamins, particularly rely on water for their absorption into the bloodstream. Adequate hydration ensures that these essential nutrients are effectively absorbed and utilized by the body.

Furthermore, water is crucial in the formation and passage of stool. Adequate hydration helps keep the stool soft, promoting regular bowel movements and preventing constipation. A well-hydrated digestive system also reduces the risk of other digestive discomforts like bloating, gas, and acid reflux.

Skin Health

The health and appearance of the skin are profoundly influenced by hydration levels. Water is a key element in maintaining skin elasticity, suppleness, and overall health.

Hydrated skin is more resilient against environmental stressors such as pollution, UV rays, and extreme temperatures. It is less prone to irritation, sensitivities, and dryness. Proper hydration helps the skin retain its moisture balance, which is essential for maintaining its protective barrier.

The hydration of skin cells plays a role in giving the skin a healthy, radiant glow. Well-hydrated skin appears more plump and vibrant, reducing the appearance of fine lines and wrinkles.

While staying hydrated alone cannot reverse the aging process, it can support overall skin health and may slow down the appearance of some aging signs. Consistent and adequate hydration can help maintain skin elasticity and reduce the likelihood of developing dry, flaky skin.

Energy and Vitality

Hydration is closely linked to overall energy levels and vitality. Water is critical for the body's metabolic processes, including energy production. Dehydration, even in its mildest forms, can have a significant impact on physical and cognitive performance.

Adequate hydration is essential for optimal brain function. The brain relies on sufficient hydration to maintain concentration, alertness, and short-term memory. Even mild dehydration can impair cognitive functions, leading to difficulties in focusing, problem-solving, and decision-making.

In terms of physical performance, water plays a vital role in transporting oxygen and nutrients to muscle tissues. This ensures that muscles function efficiently during physical activity. Adequate hydration can enhance endurance and strength, reduce the likelihood of cramps and fatigue, and aid in quicker recovery post-exercise.

The benefits of adequate hydration extend across various aspects of health – from digestive and skin health to cognitive function and physical performance. Maintaining optimal hydration levels is a simple yet effective way to support overall health, enhance vitality, and improve quality of life.

Understanding Dehydration

Dehydration is a condition that arises when the body loses more water than it consumes, leading to a disruption in the balance of salts and sugars in the blood. This imbalance can significantly affect the body's normal functioning. Understanding dehydration is crucial because even mild dehydration can impact the body's operations, while chronic dehydration can lead to more serious health consequences.

Dehydration affects the body in several ways. The body's cells and organs depend on water to function effectively. Without enough water, they can struggle to carry out their normal activities, leading to various health issues.

Consequences of Chronic Dehydration

Chronic dehydration, where the body is consistently lacking adequate water over a prolonged period, can have severe impacts on health:

- **Kidney Function**: The kidneys play a crucial role in filtering waste products and excess fluids from the blood. Adequate hydration is essential for this process. Chronic dehydration can lead to the development of kidney stones and other urinary tract problems.
- **Cardiovascular Health**: Dehydration affects the balance of electrolytes in the body, which are crucial for muscle function, including the heart. An imbalance can lead to an irregular heartbeat and other cardiovascular complications. Additionally, dehydration can cause a decrease in blood volume, making it harder for the heart to maintain adequate blood flow.
- **Digestive Issues**: Water is essential for healthy digestion. It helps in the breakdown of food and absorption of nutrients. Chronic dehydration can lead to constipation, as the body tries to conserve water by extracting more from waste, which can also increase the risk of acid reflux and other digestive disorders.

Recognizing the Signs of Dehydration

Early recognition of dehydration is important to prevent its negative effects. The common signs include:

- **Thirst and Dry Mouth**: Thirst is a primary indicator of dehydration. However, it is not always the most accurate, as dehydration can occur before we feel thirsty. A dry or sticky mouth is also a common sign.

- **Urine Output and Color**: One of the most reliable indicators of hydration is urine color. Dark-colored urine and decreased urine output are strong signs of dehydration.
- **Fatigue and Headache**: These symptoms can be among the first signs of dehydration. If dehydration continues, it can lead to more severe symptoms like dizziness, confusion, and in extreme cases, fainting.

It is essential to recognize these signs early and increase water intake accordingly. Consistently staying hydrated helps maintain the balance of bodily fluids, ensuring that the body functions optimally. This is particularly important in hot weather, during physical activity, or when unwell, as these conditions can increase the risk of dehydration.

The Hydration Equation: How Much Water Do We Need?

The "8x8 rule" (eight 8-ounce glasses of water a day) is a common guideline, but individual hydration needs can vary greatly based on factors like age, gender, climate, activity level, and overall health. A more personalized approach involves listening to your body and adjusting water intake accordingly.

Hydration Strategies for Optimal Health

Hydration is a fundamental aspect of maintaining optimal health. Achieving proper hydration involves more than just drinking water; it requires a holistic approach that integrates various hydration-friendly practices into daily life. These strategies ensure that the body receives and retains the right amount of fluids it needs to function effectively.

Water Intake Throughout the Day

One of the key strategies for maintaining hydration is ensuring regular and consistent water intake throughout the day. This practice helps maintain a constant level of hydration, which is essential for various bodily functions.

Having a water bottle handy is a practical way to remind yourself to drink water regularly. It provides a visual cue and makes it more convenient to hydrate, especially when you are on the go.

In our busy routines, it's easy to forget to drink water. Setting reminders on your phone or computer can be an effective way to ensure you're drinking water at regular intervals throughout the day.

Incorporating hydration into daily habits can also help. For example, drinking a glass of water first thing in the morning, with each meal, and before bedtime can create a routine that ensures adequate water intake.

Hydrating Foods

In addition to drinking water, consuming foods with high water content can significantly contribute to overall hydration. Many fruits and vegetables are rich in water and provide the added benefit of essential vitamins and minerals.
Foods like cucumbers, lettuce, watermelon, and oranges are high in water content. Including these in your meals and snacks can boost hydration.

Consuming broths, soups, and other liquid-based foods is another effective way to increase water intake, especially in cooler weather when you might not feel like drinking cold water.

Reducing the intake of caffeine and alcohol, which can have diuretic effects, is also important. If consuming these beverages, it's beneficial to balance them with additional water intake.

Hydration in Different Climates and Activities

Hydration needs can vary significantly based on the climate and the type of activities one engages in. Different environments and physical exertions require different hydration strategies.

In hot and humid conditions, the body loses more water through sweat. Increasing water intake is crucial in these environments to prevent dehydration. Although you might not feel as thirsty in cold weather, the body still loses water through respiratory heat loss. It's important to maintain regular hydration habits even in colder conditions.

It's essential to hydrate before, during, and after physical activities. This helps maintain optimal performance and aids in recovery. Activities like hiking, running, or sports in outdoor settings, especially in the sun, increase the need for hydration. Carrying a water bottle and taking frequent breaks for hydration is advisable.

During prolonged exercise, especially in hot weather, replacing electrolytes lost through sweat is important. Sports drinks or electrolyte supplements can be beneficial in these scenarios.

Effectively monitoring and adjusting hydration levels according to daily routines, climatic conditions, and physical activities is fundamental for good health. By implementing strategies like regular water intake, monitoring urine color, and adjusting hydration based on environmental and activity factors, one can maintain optimal hydration levels, contributing to overall well-being and health.

Overcoming Barriers to Adequate Hydration

Ensuring adequate hydration is an essential aspect of maintaining health and well-being. However, many people find it challenging to drink enough fluids each day. Overcoming the barriers to proper hydration is critical in establishing and maintaining healthy hydration habits.

Habit Formation

Forming a habit of regular water intake can be a challenge, but there are several strategies that can help:
- **Setting Reminders**: Using phone alarms or apps specifically designed for hydration can remind you to drink water at regular intervals.
- **Associating with Daily Activities**: Linking water intake with routine activities, such as drinking a glass of water before each meal or after bathroom breaks, can help establish a consistent habit.

- **Visibility and Accessibility**: Keeping a water bottle visible and within reach during the day, whether at work or home, encourages more frequent sips.

Building a habit takes time, and integrating these small steps into daily life can gradually lead to an increase in water consumption.

Flavoring Water

For those who don't enjoy the taste of plain water, adding natural flavors can make it more appealing:

- **Fruit Infusions**: Adding slices of fruits like lemon, lime, berries, or cucumber to water can infuse it with flavor without adding significant calories or sugar.
- **Herbs and Spices**: Herbs like mint, basil, or ginger can also add a refreshing twist to water.
- **Carbonation**: For those who prefer fizzy drinks, sparkling water can be a hydrating alternative, and it can also be flavored with fruit or herbs.

These simple additions can make water more enjoyable and increase the likelihood of regular consumption.

Hydration and Lifestyle

Incorporating hydration into various lifestyles requires personalized strategies:

- **At Work**: Keeping a water bottle at your desk and taking regular water breaks can help. If you're in a job that doesn't allow for easy access to water, plan to hydrate before and after work and during breaks.
- **While Traveling**: Carrying a reusable water bottle can ensure you have access to water during trips. In environments where water quality is a concern, opting for bottled water is advisable.
- **During Exercise**: Athletes or those engaging in physical activity should adjust their water intake to account for increased loss of fluids through sweat. Sports drinks with electrolytes can be beneficial during extended periods of intense exercise.

It's important to adapt hydration strategies to fit individual needs and routines. By overcoming these barriers and making hydration a part of daily life, individuals can significantly improve their overall health and well-being. Adequate hydration supports physical functions, enhances mental performance, and can contribute to a healthier lifestyle overall.

Conclusion

In conclusion, hydration is a fundamental aspect of health and vitality. It affects every cell and system in our body and is essential for maintaining optimal physical and mental function. This chapter has highlighted the importance of water in our lives, the impact of dehydration, and practical ways to ensure adequate hydration. By understanding and applying these principles, you can significantly enhance your overall health, energy levels, and well-being.

Remember, hydration is not a one-size-fits-all approach. It's about listening to your body, being mindful of your environment and activities, and making hydration an enjoyable and integral part of your daily routine. Embrace the power of water – the essence of life – and let it flow through every aspect of your journey towards health and vitality.

Chapter 5: Stress Management

Navigating the Storms: Embracing Calm in Chaos

In today's fast-paced world, managing stress is not just a luxury but a necessity for maintaining mental and physical health. Stress, while a natural response to life's challenges, can become debilitating if not managed effectively. This section explores the art of stress management and how techniques like meditation, yoga, and engaging in relaxing hobbies can serve as vital tools in maintaining calm amidst chaos.

Understanding Stress

Stress is the body's reaction to any change that requires an adjustment or response. It can be triggered by a variety of external factors, from work pressures to personal relationships, or internal factors, like health concerns or pessimistic thoughts.

While short-term (acute) stress can be motivational and improve performance, chronic (long-term) stress can be detrimental to health. Chronic stress can contribute to various health issues, including mental health disorders like anxiety and depression, cardiovascular diseases, obesity, and gastrointestinal problems.

Understanding the triggers and signs of stress is the first step in managing it. Common signs of stress include irritability, fatigue, difficulty sleeping, and changes in appetite. By recognizing these signs early, individuals can take steps to manage stress before it becomes overwhelming.

The Physiology of Stress

The body's stress response, often referred to as the "fight or flight" response, involves a series of physiological changes. The adrenal glands release hormones like adrenaline and cortisol, which prepare the body to face a perceived threat. These hormones increase heart rate, elevate blood pressure, and boost energy supplies.

This response is crucial for survival in acute situations. However, in today's world, chronic activation of this stress response can lead to physical and mental health problems. Continuous exposure to cortisol and other stress hormones can increase the risk of health issues like heart disease, diabetes, and mental disorders.

Techniques for Managing Stress

To counteract the effects of stress, several techniques can be employed:

- **Meditation**: Meditation, particularly mindfulness meditation, has been shown to reduce stress and anxiety. It involves focusing the mind on the present moment, which can help break the cycle of stress-related thoughts.
- **Yoga**: Combining physical postures, breath control, and meditation, yoga can be an effective stress-reliever. It not only aids in relaxation but also improves physical strength and flexibility.
- **Relaxing Hobbies**: Engaging in hobbies or activities that bring joy can be a powerful stress-reliever. Whether it's

reading, gardening, painting, or playing music, hobbies provide a break from stress and contribute to overall well-being.

The Art of Meditation

Meditation is a practice that dates back thousands of years, deeply rooted in various cultural and religious traditions. In recent times, it has gained popularity in the western world as a stress management and self-improvement tool. The essence of meditation lies in focusing and quieting the mind, which leads to a heightened state of awareness and inner calm.

Benefits of Meditation

Regular meditation has been shown have the benefits of:

1. **Stress Reduction**: One of the most known benefits of meditation is stress reduction. Regular meditation helps in lowering the levels of cortisol, the stress hormone, thereby reducing the physical and emotional symptoms of stress. This can include alleviating symptoms related to stress-related conditions like irritable bowel syndrome or PTSD.

2. **Anxiety Control**: Meditation helps in managing anxiety by quieting the overactive mind. Practices like mindfulness meditation train individuals to focus their attention on the present moment, reducing the tendency to ruminate on anxious thoughts.

3. **Emotional Health and Well-being**: Meditation can lead to an improved self-image and a more positive outlook on life. Mindfulness and other meditation forms can decrease depressive symptoms, leading to improved overall emotional health.

4. **Enhanced Self-Awareness**: Certain forms of meditation, like self-inquiry or mindfulness, help in developing a deeper understanding of oneself. This can lead to greater self-compassion and an understanding of personal patterns and habits.

5. **Improved Attention and Concentration**: Regular meditation practice enhances the ability to sustain attention and concentrate. This can translate to better performance in

tasks requiring focus and can be particularly beneficial in work and academic settings.

6. **Health Benefits**: Meditation has been linked to a variety of health benefits. It can help in managing symptoms of conditions like heart disease and high blood pressure by promoting relaxation and stress reduction. Additionally, meditation can improve sleep patterns, which is crucial for overall health.

Practicing Meditation

Meditation can be practiced in various forms, and finding the right fit is crucial. Three types of meditation are:

- **Mindfulness Meditation**: Involves paying attention to thoughts and feelings without judgment and focusing on the present moment.
- **Guided Meditation**: Led by a guide or teacher, this form uses visualization or imagery to achieve a state of relaxation.
- **Mantra Meditation**: Involves repeating a calming word, thought, or phrase to prevent distracting thoughts.

The key to effective meditation is consistency. Regular practice, even for a few minutes daily, can significantly enhance its benefits. It's also important to create a conducive environment for meditation - a quiet space, comfortable posture, and an open, non-judgmental mindset.

By integrating meditation into daily life, individuals can enjoy a myriad of benefits ranging from improved mental health and emotional well-being to enhanced physical health and cognitive function. Meditation not only helps in navigating the challenges of modern life with greater calm but also enhances overall life satisfaction and well-being.

The Harmony of Yoga

Yoga, a practice that originated in ancient India, has evolved over thousands of years into a comprehensive system of physical and mental disciplines. Far more than just a form of exercise, yoga is a holistic approach that integrates physical postures, controlled breathing, and meditation or relaxation. It aims to harmonize the body with the mind, fostering a sense of well-being and balance.

Yoga for Stress Relief

Yoga is renowned for its ability to relieve stress and promote relaxation, making it an invaluable tool in today's fast-paced world. The practice offers several mechanisms for stress reduction:

1. **Physical Postures (Asanas)**: Yoga asanas are designed to strengthen, stretch, and balance the body. By focusing on posture and alignment, yoga practice can release physical tension, particularly in areas like the neck, shoulders, and back where stress often accumulates. The physical activity also stimulates the release of endorphins, the body's natural mood elevators and painkillers.

2. **Breathing Techniques (Pranayama)**: Controlled breathing is a central element of yoga that helps regulate the nervous system. Pranayama practices can shift the body's balance from the sympathetic nervous system (responsible for the fight-or-flight response) to the parasympathetic nervous system, which promotes relaxation and healing.

3. **Meditation and Mindfulness**: Many yoga practices incorporate meditation or mindfulness, which helps quiet the mind and reduce stress. This aspect of yoga encourages a focus on the present moment and can lead to a reduction in the kind of rumination and worry that fuels stress and anxiety.

4. **Improvement in Overall Health**: Regular yoga practice can lead to improvements in various aspects of physical health, including cardiovascular fitness, flexibility, strength, and balance. These physical benefits, in turn, can contribute to a reduction in stress-related physical symptoms, such as headaches, muscle tension, and insomnia.

Integrating Yoga into Your Life

Incorporating yoga into daily life can be simple and does not necessarily require intensive or prolonged sessions. Even short, regular practices can yield significant benefits. The key is consistency and mindfulness.

- **Adaptability to Fitness Levels**: Yoga can be modified to suit any fitness level, making it accessible to virtually everyone, regardless of age, fitness, or health status.
- **Variety of Styles**: There are many different styles of yoga, from gentle and restorative to vigorous and challenging. This variety ensures that individuals can find a style that resonates with their personal needs and preferences.
- **Convenience**: Yoga can be practiced almost anywhere, from a studio to the comfort of one's home. Numerous online resources and apps make it easy to find guided practices for all skill levels.

By integrating yoga into daily routines, individuals can experience reduced stress, enhanced physical health, and greater mental clarity. It is a versatile practice that not only helps in coping with the stresses of modern life but also fosters a deeper sense of connection to oneself.

Engaging in Relaxing Hobbies

Hobbies, often perceived as leisure activities or pastimes, play a significant role in enhancing mental health and overall well-being. They provide an essential break from the routine stresses of life, offering a unique combination of relaxation and engagement that can rejuvenate both mind and body. Hobbies can offer:

The Power of Hobbies

Engaging in hobbies can lower stress levels, improve mood, and provide a sense of accomplishment. Whether it's gardening, painting, playing a musical instrument, or crafting, hobbies offer a valuable opportunity for self-expression and relaxation.

Engaging in hobbies is an effective way to reduce stress. Activities that you find enjoyable and fulfilling can shift focus away from stressors and provide a mental break. This shift can lower cortisol levels, the body's primary stress hormone, and promote feelings of calm and relaxation.

Hobbies have the power to boost mood by engaging in activities that bring joy and satisfaction. This positive engagement stimulates the release of neurotransmitters like dopamine and serotonin, which are associated with feelings of happiness and well-being.

Many hobbies, such as crafting, gardening, or learning a musical instrument, provide tangible results. This outcome, whether it's a finished piece of art, a well-tended garden, or a new song learned, can give a strong sense of accomplishment and pride, further enhancing self-esteem and confidence.

Hobbies often involve learning new skills, problem-solving, and creativity, which keep the brain active and engaged. This mental stimulation is essential for maintaining cognitive health, especially as one ages, and can be a protective factor against cognitive decline.

Many hobbies can lead to social interactions, whether it's joining a club, attending classes, or sharing your hobbies online. These social connections can provide support, enhance feelings of belonging, and contribute to an overall sense of community.

Finding Your Hobby

To fully reap the benefits of engaging in hobbies, it's important to choose activities that resonate personally. Here are some tips for finding the right hobby:

- **Personal Enjoyment and Interests**: Reflect on what activities you enjoy, what interests you, or what you've always wanted to try. Your hobby should be something you look forward to and enjoy doing.
- **Experimentation**: Don't be afraid to try new things. Sometimes it takes a few attempts to find the right hobby that clicks.
- **Non-Competitive Nature**: Choose hobbies that are relaxing and non-competitive, as the goal is relaxation and enjoyment, not stress or pressure to perform.
- **Balance**: Your hobby shouldn't feel like a chore or another item on your to-do list. It should be a pleasurable and relaxing activity that you can do at your own pace.
- **Accessibility and Affordability**: Consider how easily you can engage in the hobby. Some hobbies require little to no

equipment, while others might require a more significant investment.

Incorporating hobbies into your routine can significantly enhance your quality of life. They offer a fun and effective way to reduce stress, improve mood, boost creativity, and provide a sense of accomplishment. By dedicating time to hobbies, you create a valuable space for personal growth, relaxation, and joy, which are essential components of a healthy life.

Holistic Stress Management

Holistic stress management recognizes that effectively dealing with stress involves a comprehensive approach, addressing not just the symptoms but the root causes and various aspects of an individual's life. It's about creating a lifestyle that supports well-being and resilience against the challenges and pressures of life.

Balancing Life and Work

Achieving a balance between work and personal life is crucial for stress management. Here are some strategies to help create that balance:

1. **Setting Boundaries**: Establish clear boundaries between work and personal time. This might mean setting specific work hours and sticking to them, or ensuring that work doesn't encroach on personal time and activities.

2. **Prioritization and Time Management**: Learn to prioritize tasks based on importance and urgency. Effective time management can reduce the feeling of being overwhelmed and help ensure that both work and personal life receive adequate attention.

3. **Leisure and Relaxation**: It's important to set aside time for hobbies, relaxation, and leisure activities. This downtime is essential for mental and emotional well-being.

4. **Mindfulness and Presence**: Practice being present in whatever you are doing, whether it's a work task or spending time with family. Mindfulness can enhance the quality of both work and personal interactions.

Balancing work and life demands can significantly reduce stress levels and improve overall quality of life. It ensures that personal health and relationships are not neglected in the pursuit of professional success.

Healthy Lifestyle Choices

Adopting healthy lifestyle choices plays a fundamental role in managing stress:

1. **Balanced Diet**: Eating a balanced diet rich in fruits, vegetables, whole grains, lean protein, and healthy fats can provide the necessary nutrients for the body and brain to handle stress more effectively.
2. **Regular Exercise**: Physical activity is a proven stress reliever. It not only boosts physical health but also releases endorphins, the body's natural mood elevators.
3. **Adequate Sleep**: Getting enough sleep is crucial in managing stress. Sleep is a time when the body and mind can rest and recover from the day's activities and stressors.

Incorporating these healthy habits into daily life can enhance the body's ability to cope with stress, improve overall health, and lead to a more balanced and fulfilling life.

Social Connections

Having strong social connections is a powerful way to combat stress:

1. **Support Network**: A supportive network of family and friends provides a sense of belonging and security. Sharing concerns or troubles with trusted individuals can provide relief, perspective, and solutions.
2. **Enjoying Social Activities**: Engaging in social activities, whether it's a hobby, sport, or community involvement, can provide a much-needed break from stress.
3. **Emotional Support**: Having people to turn to in times of stress can provide emotional support and reduce feelings of isolation.

Strengthening social connections and ensuring a supportive network can greatly diminish the impact of stress, enhancing overall emotional and mental well-being.

Conclusion

In conclusion, managing stress is an integral part of leading a healthy and balanced life. It's about finding your calm in the chaos through various techniques like meditation, yoga, and engaging in relaxing hobbies. By understanding stress and integrating these practices into your daily life, you can navigate life's challenges with greater ease and resilience.

Remember, stress management is a journey, not a destination. It's about continual learning and adaptation, finding what works for you, and being kind to yourself in the process. By embracing these practices, you can not only manage stress but also enhance your overall well-being and quality of life.

Chapter 6: Avoid Smoking and Limit Alcohol

Steering Clear of Harm: A Journey Towards Healthier Habits

The path to wellness involves not only adopting healthy habits but also relinquishing harmful ones. Two of the most significant health challenges many face are smoking and excessive alcohol consumption. Both of these habits pose serious risks to health and well-being and overcoming them can dramatically improve one's quality of life.

Understanding the Impact

The Harms of Smoking

Smoking is one of the leading causes of preventable death globally. It's a major risk factor for numerous diseases, including lung cancer, heart disease, stroke, and chronic obstructive pulmonary disease (COPD). The smoke from cigarettes contains a lethal mix of over 7,000 chemicals, many of which are toxic and can cause damage to nearly every organ in the body. The harms of smoking may be summarized as:

1. **Widespread Health Risks**: Smoking is a primary cause of several preventable diseases. It significantly increases the risk of lung cancer, heart disease, stroke, and chronic obstructive pulmonary disease (COPD). Nicotine, the

addictive substance in cigarettes, contributes to the development of heart disease by increasing blood pressure and heart rate.

2. **Toxic Chemicals**: Cigarette smoke contains over 7,000 chemicals, many of which are toxic. These chemicals can damage nearly every organ in the body. Besides the lungs, smoking can damage the heart, blood vessels, reproductive organs, mouth, skin, eyes, and bones.

3. **Secondhand Smoke Risks**: Non-smokers exposed to secondhand smoke are at risk for many of the same diseases as smokers, including heart disease and lung cancer. This makes smoking not just a personal health issue but also a public health concern.

4. **Addiction and Dependency**: Nicotine is highly addictive, making quitting smoking a significant challenge for many. This addiction is not just physical but also psychological, often tied to routines and emotional states.

Alcohol and Health

While moderate alcohol consumption can have some health benefits for certain individuals, excessive intake is a major health hazard. These risks may be:

1. **Risks of Excessive Consumption**: While moderate alcohol consumption can be part of a healthy lifestyle for some people, excessive drinking is a major health risk. It can lead to liver diseases such as cirrhosis, increase the risk of various cancers, including breast and liver cancer, and contribute to heart health problems like high blood pressure and cardiomyopathy.

2. **Mental Health Concerns**: Excessive alcohol use can exacerbate mental health issues like depression and anxiety. It can also impair judgment and coordination, leading to accidents and injuries.

3. **Alcohol Use Disorder (AUD)**: AUD is a medical condition characterized by an inability to stop or control alcohol use despite social, occupational, or health consequences. It's a

chronic brain disease that requires medical treatment and support.

The Path to Quitting Smoking

Quitting smoking is often described as a journey rather than a destination. It's a process that embodies commitment and a willingness to overcome one of the most challenging addictions. The process of quitting smoking is as much about breaking a physical addiction as it is about transforming a deeply ingrained habit.

Understanding Addiction

Understanding the nature of nicotine addiction is crucial in the journey to quit smoking. Nicotine creates a complex addiction that is both physical and psychological. Physically, the body becomes dependent on the nicotine that cigarettes provide. Psychologically, smoking becomes a coping mechanism for stress, boredom, or social situations. Nicotine's effects on brain chemistry make quitting smoking particularly challenging, as it impacts mood, concentration, and stress levels.

Strategies for Quitting

Several strategies can aid in the process of quitting smoking, each addressing different aspects of the addiction:

1. **Nicotine Replacement Therapy (NRT)**: NRT provides a lower dose of nicotine without the harmful chemicals found in cigarettes. This can ease the withdrawal symptoms and cravings that often accompany quitting.
2. **Prescription Medications**: Medications like bupropion and varenicline can help reduce cravings and withdrawal symptoms. These medications work on the brain to lessen the pleasurable effects of nicotine.
3. **Behavioral Therapy**: Behavioral therapy, including counseling and support groups, offers a platform for sharing experiences and strategies. It also provides psychological tools to deal with cravings and triggers.
4. **Setting a Quit Date**: Choosing a specific date to quit smoking gives a clear goal and allows for mental and

physical preparation. It can also create a sense of accountability and commitment.

5. **Understanding Triggers**: Recognizing situations that trigger the urge to smoke and finding ways to avoid or cope with them is a crucial part of quitting. This may involve changing daily routines or finding new ways to manage stress.

Moderating Alcohol Intake

Moderating alcohol intake can be an essential step towards better health. For many, it requires a deeper understanding of their relationship with alcohol and the implementation of practical strategies to maintain control over their drinking habits.

Assessing Drinking Habits

The journey to moderate alcohol intake starts with a self-assessment to understand personal drinking patterns and the underlying reasons behind them. This introspection can reveal whether alcohol is being used as a coping mechanism for stress, social anxiety, or out of habit.

Strategies for Moderation

Adopting effective strategies is key to successfully moderating alcohol intake:

1. **Setting Limits**: Pre-determining the number of drinks and adhering to this limit can help maintain control over alcohol consumption.
2. **Mindful Drinking**: Being fully present and mindful while drinking can increase the enjoyment of each drink, reducing the impulse to drink excessively.
3. **Alternate with Non-Alcoholic Drinks**: Alternating alcoholic beverages with water or non-alcoholic drinks can help reduce overall alcohol intake. This also aids in staying hydrated and can reduce the effects of alcohol.
4. **Seek Support**: For some, professional help or support groups may be necessary. These resources can provide guidance, strategies, and encouragement to those struggling with moderation.

Quitting smoking and moderating alcohol intake are challenging but crucial steps towards a healthier life. These actions not only reduce the risk of various diseases but also improve overall quality of life, mental health, and physical well-being. The journey requires a comprehensive approach, combining medical, psychological, and personal strategies tailored to individual needs and situations.

Building a Support System

Embarking on a journey to quit smoking or reduce alcohol intake is a significant endeavor, one that can be made more manageable and effective with a robust support system. The role of a support network cannot be overstated in its importance for providing encouragement, advice, and a sense of accountability, all of which are crucial elements in overcoming addiction or changing lifestyle habits.

The composition of a support system can be diverse, including family members, friends, healthcare professionals, and peers who are on a similar journey. Family and friends can offer emotional support, understanding, and motivation, particularly on challenging days. Healthcare professionals, such as doctors and counselors, provide expert advice, treatment options, and can track your progress, offering professional guidance tailored to your specific needs.

In addition to emotional and professional support, peer support plays a unique and powerful role. Engaging with individuals who are going through similar experiences can provide a sense of camaraderie and mutual understanding. It can be incredibly motivating and reassuring to share experiences, challenges, and successes with peers who empathize with your journey.

Engaging with Community Resources

Community resources are a vital component of a comprehensive approach to quitting smoking or reducing alcohol intake. These resources offer support and information and often serve as a bridge between personal effort and professional medical help.

Local health centers, community organizations, and non-profits often host support groups and therapy sessions, providing a platform for people to come together and share their experiences. These groups can offer a sense of belonging, reduce feelings of isolation, and provide peer support. Additionally, many communities provide educational materials and workshops that can increase awareness about the health impacts of smoking and excessive drinking and offer strategies for overcoming these habits.

These community resources are typically run or overseen by professionals who have a deep understanding of the challenges associated with quitting smoking or reducing alcohol intake. They can provide valuable guidance and support tailored to the specific needs of the community they serve.

Online and Digital Support

In today's digital age, online resources and apps have become increasingly important in providing support for those looking to quit smoking or reduce alcohol intake. The internet offers a wealth of information, including tips, strategies, and personal stories, accessible from anywhere at any time.

There are numerous apps designed to help individuals quit smoking or control their alcohol intake. These digital tools often include features like tracking progress, setting goals, and providing reminders and motivational messages. Some apps also offer community features, allowing users to connect with others on similar journeys, share experiences, and offer mutual support.

The convenience and accessibility of online resources and digital tools mean that support is available right at your fingertips. This can be particularly beneficial for those who may not have access to in-person resources or who prefer the privacy and anonymity that online platforms can offer.

In conclusion, building a support system, engaging with community resources, and utilizing online and digital tools are all effective strategies for those seeking to quit smoking or moderate their alcohol intake. These resources provide varied forms of support, from emotional and social to informational and practical, all of which contribute significantly to the journey towards a healthier life. Having a robust support system in place can greatly increase the chances of successfully overcoming addiction and maintaining long-term health improvements.

Dealing with Relapse

Relapse is often a part of the journey toward quitting smoking or reducing alcohol intake. It's common to experience setbacks, but it's important to understand that these are not failures, but rather a part of the process. Recognizing this can help maintain motivation and resilience.

When someone trying to quit smoking or reduce alcohol consumption experiences a relapse, it's crucial not to view it as a complete derailment of progress. Instead, it can be seen as an opportunity to learn and grow. Understanding the circumstances or triggers that led to the relapse is key. This might involve identifying specific stressors, social situations, or emotional states that contributed to the setback. By recognizing these triggers, individuals can develop more effective coping strategies to prevent future relapses.

Moreover, maintaining a long-term perspective is essential. A relapse does not erase all the progress made. It's important to remember the reasons for starting this journey and to acknowledge the benefits already experienced from previous efforts.

Learning from Relapses

Each relapse carries valuable lessons. By reflecting on what led to the relapse, individuals can gain insights into their behaviors and triggers. This reflection process can involve asking questions like what was happening just before the relapse, what feelings or thoughts were present, and what could have been done differently.

Understanding these factors can help in modifying behavior and strategies to better handle similar situations in the future. It may also be helpful to discuss the relapse with a healthcare provider, therapist, or support group to gain additional perspectives and advice.

Staying Committed

Staying committed to the goal of quitting smoking or reducing alcohol intake is crucial, especially after a relapse. This commitment involves continuously reminding oneself of the reasons for starting this journey – whether it's for health, family, or personal well-being.

Recommitting to the goal might mean revisiting and possibly revising the plan to quit smoking or reduce alcohol. It could involve trying different strategies, seeking additional support, or setting new, more achievable goals. The key is to keep moving forward, using the relapse as a stepping stone rather than a stumbling block.

Physical Health Improvements

When someone quits smoking, the body begins to heal almost immediately. The heart rate and blood pressure drop within minutes to hours, the carbon monoxide level in the blood drops to normal within a day, and the risk of heart disease halves within a year. Over time, the risk of lung cancer and other respiratory diseases also significantly decreases.

Reducing alcohol consumption has immediate effects as well, such as improved sleep quality and higher energy levels. Over time, it can lead to weight loss, reduced liver fat, and a lower risk of chronic diseases like liver disease and some types of cancer.

Mental and Emotional Benefits

Beyond the physical health benefits, quitting smoking and reducing alcohol intake can significantly improve mental health and emotional well-being. Many individuals report reduced anxiety and stress, better mood regulation, and an overall increase in mental clarity. The sense of achievement and control over one's life that comes from successfully making these changes can also boost self-esteem and overall life satisfaction.

In conclusion, dealing with relapse is a critical aspect of the journey to quit smoking and reduce alcohol intake. Understanding that relapses can occur and learning from them can strengthen future attempts. The commitment to this journey is underpinned by the numerous benefits, including improved physical health and enhanced mental and emotional well-being.

Conclusion

In conclusion, while the journey to quit smoking and reduce alcohol intake is challenging, it is immensely rewarding. It not only improves physical health but also enhances mental and emotional well-being. This chapter has provided insights into the impact of these habits, practical strategies to overcome them, and the importance of a support system.

Remember, every step towards reducing these harmful habits is a step towards a healthier, more vibrant life. The journey may be long and winding, but it leads to a destination of improved health and well-being.

Chapter 7: Regular Health Check-ups

The Proactive Path: Embracing Preventive Healthcare

In the realm of personal health, a proactive approach through preventive healthcare is invaluable. This approach is about taking charge of your health by regularly engaging in activities and check-ups that aim to prevent diseases or catch them early when they are more treatable. Embracing preventive healthcare transforms the way we view and manage our health, shifting the focus from reacting to health problems to actively preventing them.

Understanding Preventive Healthcare

Preventive healthcare is the practice of caring for your health proactively, with an emphasis on the prevention of diseases and maintenance of well-being. This approach encompasses a wide range of practices, from lifestyle changes and regular exercise to vaccinations and regular health screenings.

The cornerstone of preventive healthcare is the early detection and prevention of diseases. Regular screenings and medical check-ups are designed to identify risk factors and early signs of diseases, such as cancer, diabetes, or heart disease, at a stage when they are most treatable. Early detection often means more effective and less invasive treatment, and in many cases, it can lead to better health outcomes.

Beyond disease detection, preventive healthcare also includes steps to avoid the development of health issues in the first place. This involves adopting a healthy lifestyle, including balanced nutrition, regular physical activity, sufficient sleep, and managing stress. It also involves being informed about your health and understanding how to maintain it.

The Role of Regular Check-ups

Regular health check-ups are a fundamental aspect of preventive healthcare. They provide a baseline of one's health and are instrumental in detecting changes over time. These check-ups can vary based on age, gender, and personal health history but typically include blood tests, blood pressure checks, cholesterol levels, and other screenings as recommended by healthcare providers.

During these check-ups, healthcare professionals not only look for signs of potential health issues but also offer advice on maintaining and improving health. They can provide guidance on lifestyle changes, diet, exercise, and managing risk factors like high blood pressure or cholesterol. Regular check-ups also offer an opportunity to discuss any health concerns and get professional medical advice.

In addition to physical health check-ups, preventive healthcare also emphasizes mental health. Regular consultations with mental health professionals can be crucial in maintaining emotional well-being, especially for individuals with a history of mental health issues or those undergoing significant life stressors.

The Lifesaving Potential of Screenings

Health screenings serve as a critical element in the proactive management of health, offering a vital opportunity for the early detection of diseases such as cancer, diabetes, and heart disease. These screenings are not just routine procedures; they are potentially lifesaving tools that can significantly alter the course of one's health journey.

Screenings are particularly crucial because many health conditions and diseases, including various forms of cancer and heart disease, can develop silently and remain undetected until they reach more advanced stages. By detecting diseases in their early stages, when they are often more treatable, screenings can lead to better health outcomes. For example, early detection of cancer can increase the effectiveness of treatment, reduce the need for more aggressive therapies, and improve survival rates.

Types of Health Screenings

There are several types of health screenings, each targeting specific diseases:

1. **Cancer Screenings**: These are designed to detect cancer before symptoms appear. Tests like mammograms for breast cancer, colonoscopies for colorectal cancer, Pap smears for cervical cancer, and skin examinations for skin cancer are among the common screenings. The type of screening and its frequency depend on factors like age, gender, and family history.
2. **Cardiovascular Screenings**: These screenings are essential for detecting risk factors for heart disease and stroke. Regular blood pressure checks and cholesterol tests are simple yet effective ways to identify individuals at risk. These screenings can lead to early interventions, such as lifestyle changes or medications to manage these risk factors.
3. **Diabetes Screenings**: Blood sugar tests are used to screen for diabetes, a condition that can often be managed effectively if caught early. Regular diabetes screenings are particularly important for individuals with risk factors such as obesity, a family history of diabetes, or a history of gestational diabetes.

Integrating Check-ups into Your Lifestyle

Incorporating regular health check-ups into your lifestyle is a conscious decision to prioritize your health. It involves understanding the importance of these screenings and recognizing them as a crucial investment in your long-term well-being.

Scheduling and Planning

To effectively integrate health screenings into your life, it's important to establish a routine. This could mean scheduling annual check-ups or setting reminders for specific screenings based on your age, gender, and health history. Keeping a health calendar can be an effective way to track these appointments and ensure that they are not overlooked. This calendar can include dates for regular screenings, follow-up appointments, and any other health-related activities.

In conclusion, health screenings are an essential aspect of preventive healthcare, offering the potential to save lives by detecting diseases early. By understanding the types of screenings available and integrating them into your lifestyle, you can take a proactive stance in managing your health. This proactive approach can lead to early detection of diseases, more effective treatment, and ultimately, a healthier, longer life.

Personalized Healthcare

Personalized healthcare is a modern approach that emphasizes the unique health needs and considerations of each individual. Unlike a one-size-fits-all approach, personalized healthcare tailors medical care to the individual characteristics, needs, and preferences of patients. This approach can significantly enhance the effectiveness of care, leading to better health outcomes and a more satisfying healthcare experience.

Understanding Your Health Needs

Recognizing that every individual has unique health needs is the first step towards personalized healthcare. Several factors contribute to these unique needs:

1. **Age**: Different stages of life come with different health risks and requirements. For instance, health concerns for a child will be different from those of an elderly person.

2. **Family History**: A person's genetic background can significantly influence their risk for certain conditions, such as heart disease, diabetes, or certain types of cancer.
3. **Lifestyle Choices**: Factors like diet, exercise, smoking, and alcohol consumption play a significant role in an individual's health. Lifestyle choices can either increase or decrease the risk of various health conditions.
4. **Existing Health Conditions**: Individuals with chronic conditions such as hypertension or asthma require tailored care and management strategies.

Healthcare providers can help identify the most appropriate screenings, preventive measures, and treatments based on these factors. They can advise on lifestyle changes, screen for diseases more common in certain age groups or with specific family histories, and manage chronic conditions more effectively.

The Importance of a Trusted Healthcare Provider

Having a trusted healthcare provider is crucial in navigating the complexities of health and medical care. A healthcare provider who knows your health history, understands your concerns, and respects your preferences can provide more effective and personalized care.

Such a provider can help interpret screening results, suggest appropriate follow-up actions, and guide you through health decisions. They can also provide valuable information and education about your health, empowering you to make informed choices.

Building a Relationship with Your Provider

Developing a strong, ongoing relationship with a healthcare provider has numerous benefits. When a provider is familiar with your health history, lifestyle, and personal preferences, they can offer more nuanced and effective care. This relationship also fosters better communication, allowing you to feel more comfortable sharing concerns and asking questions.

A healthcare provider who knows you well can more easily detect changes in your health over time, leading to earlier intervention when necessary. They can also help coordinate care among specialists and other healthcare services, ensuring a more seamless healthcare experience.

In summary, personalized healthcare is a vital component of modern medical care. It takes into account the unique health needs of each individual, leading to more effective and satisfactory health outcomes. By understanding your specific health needs, building a relationship with a trusted healthcare provider, and benefiting from their personalized advice and care, you can take a more active and informed role in managing your health.

Navigating Health Anxiety

Health anxiety, especially regarding medical check-ups and screenings, is a common concern. It stems from the fear of the unknown and the potential for unfavorable diagnoses. However, understanding the role of these check-ups in preventive healthcare and building a trusting relationship with a healthcare provider can significantly alleviate these fears.

Dealing with Health Anxiety

Education and communication are key in managing health anxiety. Learning about the nature and purpose of health screenings can demystify them and reduce fear. These check-ups are not just about finding problems but are primarily focused on maintaining health and preventing illness.

Discussing concerns with a healthcare provider can also be reassuring. A good provider will take the time to explain procedures and answer questions, helping to alleviate fears and misconceptions. Remember, these screenings are proactive steps towards safeguarding your health and are conducted in a controlled, safe environment.

The Role of Lifestyle in Preventive Healthcare

Lifestyle choices, such as diet, exercise, smoking, and alcohol consumption, have a significant impact on overall health. Regular health check-ups offer an opportunity to discuss these lifestyle factors with a healthcare professional and understand their impact on your health.

Lifestyle and Screening Interplay

There is a dynamic interplay between lifestyle choices and health screenings. Screenings can identify areas where lifestyle changes are necessary, providing a tangible impetus for modification. Conversely, adopting healthier lifestyle choices can positively influence the results of future screenings, reflecting improvements in aspects like blood pressure, cholesterol levels, and body mass index.

Making informed lifestyle choices can enhance your health and potentially reduce the risk of conditions that screenings aim to detect, such as heart disease, diabetes, and certain cancers.

Overcoming Barriers to Regular Check-ups

While the importance of regular health check-ups is clear, various factors can impede their regularity. Time constraints, financial concerns, and fear of medical procedures or results are common barriers.

Addressing Common Barriers

- **Time Management**: Prioritizing health appointments in your schedule is crucial.
- **Financial Concerns**: Exploring insurance options or community health programs can make screenings more accessible.
- **Fear of Results**: Focusing on the proactive aspect of screenings can help overcome the fear of potential health issues.

Health Literacy: Understanding and Advocacy

Health literacy is vital in navigating the healthcare system and making informed decisions. Being knowledgeable about health-related matters enables you to be a more active participant in your healthcare.

Enhancing Health Literacy

Increasing your health literacy can involve educating yourself about various health topics, screenings, and potential diseases. Make it a habit to ask questions during your medical appointments and seek clarifications on any health-related issues you do not fully understand.

Being informed and proactive in your healthcare can lead to better health outcomes. It empowers you to make informed decisions and take charge of your health journey, ultimately leading to a healthier life.

The Ripple Effect of Regular Check-ups

Regular health check-ups, while primarily a personal health tool, have a wider impact that extends beyond the individual. These check-ups, often perceived as routine and personal, can actually have a profound ripple effect on families, communities, and even the broader health system. By prioritizing one's health through regular check-ups, individuals not only safeguard their well-being but also contribute positively to the health culture of their immediate and extended circles.

The concept of the ripple effect in health check-ups is rooted in the idea that individual health behaviors can influence the attitudes and actions of others. When you consistently engage in regular health screenings and check-ups, you set a precedent and a standard for health consciousness that can be influential.

Inspiring Others

Your commitment to health can serve as a powerful form of inspiration and motivation for others. Family members, friends, and even colleagues are often influenced by the health choices and practices they observe in their social circles. When they see you taking proactive steps towards maintaining your health, it can prompt them to reflect on their own health practices.

For instance, when parents prioritize their health check-ups, they not only ensure their ability to care for their family but also model healthy behavior for their children. This modeling can instill a lifelong appreciation for preventive healthcare in the next generation. Similarly, in a workplace setting, when employees observe their peers taking time for health check-ups, it can encourage a culture of health awareness and responsibility.

Moreover, regular check-ups can lead to early detection and management of health issues, which can reduce the burden on family members who might otherwise need to provide care or support in more advanced stages of illness. It also contributes to a healthier community by reducing the spread of communicable diseases, managing public health risks, and easing the load on healthcare systems.

In conclusion, the benefits of regular health check-ups extend far beyond the individual. They create a positive impact that ripples through families, communities, and the broader society. By prioritizing regular health screenings, individuals not only enhance their own well-being but also contribute to the collective health and inspire those around them to value and invest in their health. This collective effort towards preventive healthcare can lead to stronger, healthier communities and a more resilient public health system.

Conclusion

In conclusion, regular health check-ups and screenings are essential components of a wholesome life. They are proactive steps in preventive healthcare, allowing for early detection and management of potential health issues. By making these check-ups an integral part of your health regimen, you take a significant step towards maintaining and enhancing your overall well-being.

Remember, your health is your most valuable asset. Investing in regular check-ups and screenings is investing in your future, ensuring that you can lead a vibrant, healthy life. Embrace the proactive path of preventive healthcare, and let it guide you towards lasting health and vitality.

Chapter 8: Mental Health Awareness

Embracing Mental Wellness: A Journey to Inner Peace

In the pursuit of overall well-being, mental health is as significant as physical health, yet it often does not receive the same attention and care. Mental wellness is a critical aspect of our lives, influencing our thoughts, emotions, and behaviors. In this chapter, we explore the various facets of mental health, emphasizing its importance and providing guidance on nurturing mental wellness.

Understanding Mental Health

Mental health encompasses the state of our emotional, psychological, and social well-being. It is a complex and multifaceted aspect of our lives, influencing not only how we process and interpret the world around us but also how we handle stress, relate to others, and make decisions. Mental health is foundational to our daily functioning and overall quality of life.

Contrary to some misconceptions, mental health is not just about the absence of mental disorders. It is about being in a state of well-being where individuals are aware of their abilities, can manage the normal stresses of life, work productively, and contribute to their communities. This positive aspect of mental health is essential for our relationships, work, and physical health.

The Spectrum of Mental Health

Mental health is not a static condition but a spectrum that ranges from excellent mental well-being to severe mental health disorders. This spectrum is dynamic, influenced by a multitude of factors, including genetics, life experiences, and brain chemistry. Everyday stressors, interpersonal relationships, work environments, and social contexts can all impact mental health.

Recognizing the fluid nature of mental health is essential. It can fluctuate over time, with individuals experiencing periods of good mental health as well as times of mental distress or illness. This understanding is crucial for acknowledging the importance of proactive mental health care and maintenance. Just like physical health, mental health requires regular attention and can benefit significantly from preventive measures.

In summary, embracing mental wellness is a journey that involves understanding and caring for our mental health just as we do our physical health. It requires acknowledging the importance of mental well-being in our overall quality of life and understanding the dynamic nature of mental health. By doing so, we can work towards achieving a state of inner peace and well-being, enhancing our ability to live fulfilling and productive lives.

Recognizing the Importance of Mental Health

The importance of mental health in leading a fulfilling and balanced life cannot be overstated. Mental health, often overshadowed by physical health, is crucial for overall well-being and profoundly impacts every aspect of our lives.

Good mental health is more than the absence of mental disorders. It involves the capacity to enjoy life, endure challenges, and bounce back from adversities. It encompasses our emotional, psychological, and cognitive well-being and is fundamental to our capacity to think, feel, and interact with others.

When mental health is nurtured, individuals can realize their full potential, cope with the normal stresses of life, work productively, and contribute to their communities. The benefits of maintaining good mental health are extensive. It leads to improved mood and emotional regulation, reduced levels of anxiety and stress, and enhances resilience – the ability to adapt in the face of adversity.

Additionally, mental health significantly impacts physical health. Poor mental health can contribute to a range of physical ailments, from heart disease to weakened immune systems, highlighting the interconnection between the mind and body.

The Stigma of Mental Health

Despite its critical importance, mental health often faces societal stigma and misconceptions. Stigma around mental health can manifest in various forms, including societal judgment, self-stigma, or a general lack of understanding and empathy. This stigma can be debilitating, leading individuals to feel ashamed or embarrassed about their mental health conditions, which can prevent them from seeking the necessary help and support.

Breaking down these stigmas is vital for creating a supportive environment for mental health. Education plays a key role in this, helping to dispel myths and misinformation about mental health conditions. Encouraging open and honest conversations about mental health is essential in normalizing these discussions and reducing stigma.

Showing compassion and empathy towards those experiencing mental health issues is also crucial. Supportive communities and networks can provide the necessary understanding and assistance for those struggling with mental health, helping them to seek and receive help without fear of judgment or discrimination.

Mental health is a fundamental aspect of overall well-being, integral to living a balanced and fulfilling life. Recognizing its importance, addressing the challenges it faces, including stigma, and taking proactive steps to nurture mental health are crucial. A society that values and supports mental wellness is one that enables its members to thrive both mentally and physically.

Indicators of Mental Health Issues

Recognizing when to seek professional help is critical in addressing mental health issues effectively. If these signs and symptoms persist and begin to interfere significantly with day-to-day life and routines, such as impacting work performance, relationships, or overall quality of life, it's time to seek assistance. Additionally, if there's ever a point where there are thoughts of self-harm or suicide, it's crucial to seek help immediately.

Mental health issues can manifest through emotional, behavioral, and physical symptoms. It's important to be aware of these signs, both in oneself and in others:

- **Emotional Symptoms**: Prolonged sadness, irritability, or heightened emotions such as excessive fears or worries that seem disproportionate to the situation are common emotional indicators. These might manifest as feelings of hopelessness or helplessness, often without a clear cause.
- **Behavioral Changes**: Extreme mood swings that impact relationships, withdrawal from social activities, and loss of interest in hobbies previously enjoyed are significant behavioral signs. These changes might include isolating oneself, neglecting responsibilities, or a noticeable decrease in performance at work or school.
- **Physical Symptoms**: Mental health issues often have physical manifestations, such as persistent headaches, stomachaches, or other unexplained physical symptoms. Changes in appetite or sleeping patterns, whether eating or sleeping too much or too little, are also common indicators.
- **Cognitive Symptoms**: Difficulty concentrating, persistent negative thoughts, and in severe cases, thoughts of self-harm or harming others are crucial cognitive signs that should not be ignored.

When to Seek Help

Recognizing when to seek professional help is essential for effective treatment and management of mental health issues. It's important to seek assistance when:

- **Symptoms Become Overwhelming**: If the signs of mental health issues persist and start significantly interfering with daily life, such as affecting work, education, relationships, or general functioning, it's time to consider professional help.
- **Quality of Life is Affected**: When mental health symptoms reduce the overall quality of life, leading to distress, social isolation, or an inability to cope with daily challenges, professional intervention can provide necessary support and treatment.
- **Safety is a Concern**: Any thoughts or plans of self-harm or suicide are immediate red flags. In such cases, it's crucial to seek help immediately, either by contacting a mental health professional, a crisis hotline, or visiting an emergency room.

Being vigilant about the indicators of mental health issues and recognizing when to seek help are pivotal aspects of maintaining mental wellness. Addressing mental health concerns promptly can lead to more effective management and recovery, ultimately contributing to a healthier, more fulfilling life.

Strategies for Maintaining Mental Well-being

Adopting strategies to maintain mental well-being is a proactive approach that is essential for overall health. Mental well-being involves more than just the absence of mental health issues; it encompasses a positive state of emotional and psychological health where an individual can effectively handle stress, work productively, and contribute to their community.

Mindfulness and Meditation

Incorporating mindfulness and meditation into daily routines can significantly impact mental well-being. These practices are centered around cultivating a heightened state of awareness and presence.

Mindfulness involves focusing on the present moment without judgment. Mindfulness can be practiced in everyday activities like eating, walking, or even during work. By paying attention to the present, mindfulness helps break the cycle of negative thought patterns, reducing stress and anxiety. It encourages acceptance and can lead to a more profound understanding of oneself and one's reactions, fostering emotional resilience.

Meditation practices can vary, but they typically involve focused attention and deep breathing. These practices quiet the mind and can reduce stress hormone levels in the body. Regular meditation can lead to changes in the brain associated with improved emotional regulation, increased attention span, and enhanced self-awareness.

Physical Activity and Mental Health

Regular physical activity plays a crucial role in promoting mental health alongside physical health.

- **Releasing Endorphins**: Exercise, particularly aerobic activities like walking, running, and swimming, stimulates the release of endorphins, often described as the body's natural mood lifters. These chemicals in the brain improve mood and reduce the perception of pain.

- **Combating Depression and Anxiety**: Physical activity can be a powerful tool in managing depression and anxiety. It provides a distraction, allowing for a break from negative thoughts and enabling the individual to find quiet time for mental relaxation. Additionally, regular exercise can improve self-esteem and cognitive function, both of which are important for mental health.
- **Improving Sleep and Stress Management**: Exercise also contributes to better sleep quality, which is crucial for mental well-being. It can improve sleep onset and duration, as well as the quality of sleep. Moreover, physical activity is an effective stress reducer. It helps in the management of physical and mental stress, improving the body's ability to deal with existing mental tension.

Building Strong Relationships

Positive relationships are a crucial source of emotional support. They provide a safe space for expressing feelings, sharing experiences, and seeking advice. These interactions help in validating our experiences and feelings, offering reassurance and understanding.

- **Emotional Support**: Healthy relationships offer a platform for emotional expression and support. Knowing that there are people who care and are available to listen can be immensely comforting, especially during tough times. The emotional support provided by strong relationships can help mitigate feelings of loneliness and isolation.
- **Sense of Belonging**: Strong relationships contribute to a sense of belonging and connectedness. Humans are social beings, and having a sense of belonging to a community or group provides psychological comfort. It can enhance self-esteem and a sense of identity.
- **Buffer Against Mental Health Issues**: Relationships can act as a buffer against mental health issues like depression and anxiety. The support, understanding, and validation received

from relationships can help individuals navigate stressors and challenges more effectively.

- **Comfort and Relief During Difficult Times**: In times of crisis or stress, having a network of supportive relationships can offer significant comfort and relief. Whether it's coping with loss, navigating personal challenges, or enduring stressful situations, the presence and support of loved ones can be a critical factor in resilience and recovery.

Fostering and Maintaining Strong Relationships

Building and maintaining strong relationships requires effort and commitment. It involves open and honest communication, empathy, and mutual respect. It's also important to invest time and energy into relationships, participating in shared activities, and being present for the other person.

- **Active Communication**: Open and honest communication is the foundation of any strong relationship. It involves not just talking but also actively listening and trying to understand the other person's perspective.
- **Empathy and Understanding**: Showing empathy and trying to understand the feelings and experiences of others strengthens bonds and builds trust.
- **Investing Time and Effort**: Relationships thrive when time and effort are invested. This could be through regular interactions, shared experiences, or simply being there for one another in times of need.

Bilding and maintaining strong, healthy relationships are crucial for mental well-being. These relationships provide essential emotional support, a sense of belonging, and act as a buffer against various mental health challenges. By fostering open communication, empathy, and investing time and effort, individuals can build relationships that enrich their lives and enhance their mental health.

The Role of Professional Help

Professional intervention plays a critical role in effectively addressing and managing mental health issues. Mental health professionals offer specialized support that can significantly impact an individual's journey towards mental wellness. They provide expertise in therapy, counseling, or medication, tailored to the specific needs and conditions of their clients.

Mental health professionals are equipped with the training and tools necessary to diagnose, treat, and manage a wide range of mental health disorders. Their expertise allows for a comprehensive approach to treatment, which may include a combination of therapy, counseling, and medication.

- **Holistic Approach to Treatment**: Professional help often involves a holistic approach that addresses both the emotional and biochemical aspects of mental health issues. This approach can be particularly beneficial in complex or severe cases where multiple modalities of treatment are necessary.
- **Customized Treatment Plans**: Mental health professionals can create personalized treatment plans based on individual needs, histories, and specific mental health conditions. These plans may evolve over time as the individual makes progress or as their needs change.

Types of Mental Health Professionals

Navigating the world of mental health care can be overwhelming, but understanding the roles of different types of mental health professionals can help in seeking appropriate care.

- **Psychologists and Counselors**: These professionals typically focus on providing therapy and counseling. They utilize various therapeutic techniques to help individuals understand their feelings, thoughts, and behaviors, and develop coping strategies. They cannot prescribe medication.
- **Psychiatrists**: Psychiatrists are medical doctors who specialize in mental health. They are qualified to diagnose mental health conditions, prescribe and manage medication, and also provide therapy. Their medical training allows them to understand the biological as well as psychological aspects of mental disorders.

Therapy and Counseling

Therapy and counseling are pivotal elements in the treatment of mental health issues. These interventions provide a safe, confidential environment where individuals can explore their feelings, thoughts, and behaviors.

- **Safe and Confidential Space**: Therapy offers a non-judgmental space where individuals can freely discuss their issues without fear of stigma or repercussions. This environment is crucial for honest self-reflection and healing.
- **Understanding and Coping Strategies**: Through therapy, individuals can gain insights into their mental health conditions, understand patterns in their thoughts and behaviors, and develop effective coping strategies. This understanding is key to managing symptoms and improving overall mental health.
- **Support and Guidance**: Mental health professionals provide support, guidance, and validation throughout the therapeutic process. They help navigate the complexities of mental health issues, offering support in times of crisis and guiding individuals towards recovery.

Medication and Mental Health

The use of medication in managing mental health conditions is a crucial aspect of contemporary psychiatric care. For many mental health disorders, medication can play a vital role in treatment, often being necessary to manage symptoms effectively. It's important to recognize the role of medication in the broader context of mental health treatment and understand its appropriate use.

Medications for mental health, often referred to as psychotropic drugs, are designed to treat psychiatric disorders by influencing brain chemicals that affect mood and behavior. These medications can include antidepressants, anti-anxiety medications, mood stabilizers, and antipsychotics, among others.

It is imperative that mental health medications are prescribed and monitored by qualified healthcare professionals. Psychiatrists, in particular, have specialized training in managing these medications, understanding their effects, and monitoring for side effects.

Medication is often most effective when combined with other forms of treatment, such as therapy and lifestyle changes. This comprehensive approach can address the psychological, behavioral, and social aspects of mental health conditions.
Medication can be a crucial component of treatment for mental health conditions. When used under the guidance of healthcare professionals and combined with therapy and lifestyle changes, medication can significantly improve the management of symptoms and enhance the quality of life for those with mental health disorders.

Overcoming Barriers to Seeking Help

Seeking help for mental health issues is a vital step in the journey towards wellness. However, numerous barriers often prevent individuals from accessing the help they need. Understanding and actively addressing these barriers is crucial for ensuring that everyone has the opportunity to receive appropriate mental health support.

Addressing Stigma

Stigma surrounding mental health is one of the most formidable barriers to seeking help. This stigma can manifest in various ways, from societal attitudes to internalized shame, leading to reluctance in seeking help.

One effective way to combat stigma is through education and raising awareness. Understanding mental health challenges can foster empathy and support within communities. This involves openly discussing mental health issues, sharing personal stories, and engaging in public education campaigns. Such efforts help to normalize mental health struggles and break down misconceptions.

Creating environments where mental health can be openly discussed without fear of judgment or reprisal is key. This includes in workplaces, schools, families, and social circles. Open dialogues can make a significant difference in how mental health is perceived and can encourage individuals to seek help when needed.

Accessibility of Mental Health Services

Accessibility to mental health services is another major barrier. Many people struggle to access care due to various reasons, including financial constraints, geographical limitations, and a lack of available services.

Addressing the issue of accessibility includes advocating for better mental health coverage in health insurance and increased funding for mental health services. This advocacy can help make mental health care more affordable and accessible to a broader segment of the population.

Increasing the number of trained mental health professionals and expanding mental health services, especially in underserved areas, is crucial. This expansion can help reduce waiting times and make services more readily available to those in need.

The use of telehealth has emerged as a powerful tool in making mental health care more accessible. Telehealth services can be particularly beneficial for individuals in remote or underserved areas, or for those who have mobility or scheduling challenges that make in-person therapy difficult.

Overcoming barriers to seeking help for mental health issues is essential for the well-being of individuals and communities. Addressing stigma and improving the accessibility of mental health services are key steps in ensuring that everyone who needs mental health support can receive it. Through education, advocacy, and the expansion of services, we can create a more inclusive and supportive environment for mental health care.

The Impact of Lifestyle on Mental Health

The influence of lifestyle factors on mental health is profound and multifaceted. A balanced lifestyle, incorporating elements like a nutritious diet, sufficient sleep, and effective stress management, plays a significant role in enhancing mental well-being. Understanding and optimizing these aspects can lead to substantial improvements in emotional and psychological health.

Diet and Mental Health

The connection between diet and mental health is increasingly recognized as critical. What we consume not only affects our physical health but also has a direct impact on our mental state. Emerging research in the field of nutritional psychiatry suggests that diet is as important to mental health as it is to physical health. A diet that provides essential nutrients contributes significantly to the functioning of the brain and the regulation of mood.

Certain nutrients are particularly important for brain health and mood regulation. Omega-3 fatty acids, found in fatty fish, flaxseeds, and walnuts, are known for their role in brain health and cognitive function. Vitamins, such as B-vitamins and vitamin D, and minerals like magnesium and zinc, play roles in neurotransmitter function and mood regulation.

Consuming a diet that encompasses a variety of these nutrients can positively influence mental health. Incorporating a range of fruits, vegetables, whole grains, lean proteins, and healthy fats ensures a balanced intake of these essential nutrients. This kind of diet supports not only physical health but also contributes to emotional and psychological well-being.

Sleep and Mental Health

The relationship between sleep and mental health is bidirectional - poor mental health can lead to sleep problems, and conversely, poor sleep can adversely affect mental health.

Quality sleep plays a crucial role in processing emotional information and consolidating memories, both of which are vital for cognitive function and emotional regulation. Disrupted or inadequate sleep can exacerbate conditions like anxiety and depression and can impair cognitive abilities.

Establishing a regular sleep schedule is key to improving sleep quality. This includes going to bed and waking up at the same time each day to regulate the body's internal clock. Creating a comfortable and conducive sleep environment, free from distractions and conducive to relaxation, is also important. Good sleep hygiene practices, such as limiting screen time before bed, avoiding caffeine and heavy meals in the evening, and engaging in relaxing activities like reading or meditation, can significantly enhance sleep quality.

Lifestyle factors such as diet and sleep have a significant impact on mental health. A balanced diet rich in essential nutrients and healthy sleep habits are foundational in maintaining and improving mental well-being. By focusing on these aspects, individuals can greatly enhance their emotional and psychological health, leading to a better quality of life.

The Importance of Self-Care

Self-care is a vital component of mental health maintenance, playing a critical role in managing stress, enhancing well-being, and improving overall quality of life. It involves intentionally taking time for activities that nurture and rejuvenate oneself on a physical, emotional, and mental level.

Self-care is about more than just indulging in pleasurable activities; it's a holistic approach to taking care of oneself. This involves understanding and tending to your needs, setting boundaries, and making choices that enhance your long-term health and happiness.

Regular self-care can significantly impact mental health. It helps in managing stress, reducing the risk of burnout, and boosting mood. It allows for a space to process emotions, clear the mind, and reduce anxiety.

Engaging in self-care is also an act of self-compassion and empowerment. It's about recognizing your worth and taking the necessary steps to care for your well-being. This practice can lead to improved self-esteem and a more positive outlook on life.

Developing a Self-Care Routine

Creating a self-care routine involves identifying activities that bring joy, relaxation, and rejuvenation. The activities chosen can vary widely from person to person, depending on individual interests and what brings them relaxation and happiness.

Self-care activities can range from hobbies and leisure activities to simpler practices. This might include engaging in creative pursuits like painting or writing, participating in physical activities like yoga or hiking, or enjoying quiet time with activities like reading or taking a warm bath.

Spending time in nature is another valuable self-care practice. Whether it's a walk in the park, gardening, or just sitting outside, being in natural settings can have a calming effect and improve mental well-being.

The most important aspect of developing a self-care routine is personalization. It should reflect activities that you genuinely enjoy and find relaxing. It's not about what you think you should be doing, but what truly brings you peace and joy.

Incorporating self-care into your daily life requires consistency, but it's also important to be flexible. Life's demands can change, and so can your self-care needs. It's about finding a balance and adjusting your self-care practices as needed.

Self-care is an indispensable aspect of maintaining mental health. It involves taking time to engage in activities that rejuvenate and bring joy, leading to improved mental and emotional well-being. By developing a personalized and flexible self-care routine, individuals can effectively manage stress, enhance their mood, and foster overall health and happiness.

Conclusion

In conclusion, mental health is a crucial aspect of overall health and should be given equal importance as physical health. This chapter has highlighted the significance of mental well-being, the importance of recognizing mental health issues, strategies for maintaining mental health, and the role of professional help.

Remember, taking care of your mental health is not a sign of weakness but a mark of strength. It's about acknowledging your needs and taking steps to meet them. By prioritizing mental health, you not only improve your quality of life but also contribute to a healthier, more compassionate society.

Chapter 9: Maintain a Healthy Weight

Nurturing Your Body: A Balanced Approach to Weight

In a world obsessed with body image, maintaining a healthy weight is often misconstrued as striving for an ideal figure. However, the essence of a healthy weight lies in nurturing the body, ensuring its optimal functioning and longevity. This chapter explores the symbiotic relationship between a balanced diet, regular exercise, and maintaining a healthy weight, shifting the focus from aesthetic ideals to overall health and well-being.

Understanding Healthy Weight

A healthy weight is a concept that goes beyond a mere number on a scale. It's an individualized measure that varies significantly based on several factors such as age, gender, muscle mass, bone density, and overall body composition. This weight is essentially where your body functions most efficiently and with the least risk of health complications like cardiovascular diseases, diabetes, and other weight-related conditions.

The definition of a healthy weight acknowledges that weight is a highly individual matter. For instance, two people of the same height and weight might have completely different health profiles, depending on their muscle mass and bone density. Additionally, factors like genetic makeup, metabolic rate, and lifestyle play a crucial role in determining what a healthy weight means for an individual.

Beyond the Scale

Focusing solely on the scale to determine health can be misleading. Body weight alone does not distinguish between the various components that make up total body weight - fat, muscle, bone, and water. A more holistic approach considers body composition, which refers to the percentages of fat, bone, muscle, and water in the body.

Body composition is crucial because muscle tissue is denser than fat tissue. Therefore, a person with a high muscle mass might weigh more but is not necessarily less healthy. In contrast, someone might be at a 'normal' weight according to the scale but could have a higher percentage of body fat, a condition known as 'normal weight obesity' or 'skinny fat.'

The Role of a Balanced Diet

Achieving and maintaining a healthy weight is intrinsically linked to diet. A balanced diet is not about strict limitations or depriving oneself but about integrating a variety of nutrients in appropriate proportions. This balanced approach ensures that the body receives the necessary fuel to function efficiently and maintain muscle mass while managing fat levels.

Nutrient-Rich Foods

Incorporating a range of nutrient-rich foods is fundamental to a balanced diet. These foods provide the essential vitamins, minerals, and other nutrients the body needs for optimal functioning. A healthy diet should include a mix of:

- Fruits and vegetables, which are rich in vitamins, minerals, and fiber.
- Whole grains, which provide essential B vitamins and fiber.
- Lean proteins, which are crucial for muscle building and repair.
- Healthy fats, such as those found in avocados, nuts, and olive oil, which are vital for brain health and hormone production.

Mindful Eating

Mindful eating is an approach that emphasizes being fully present and engaged during eating experiences. It involves savoring each bite and paying attention to your body's hunger and fullness signals. This practice encourages a healthier relationship with food, where eating is guided by physiological cues rather than emotional triggers. Mindful eating can help prevent overeating and is conducive to maintaining a healthy weight.

In summary, understanding healthy weight involves considering a range of factors beyond the scale, including body composition and individual physiological differences. Achieving and maintaining a healthy weight is supported by a balanced diet rich in nutrient-dense foods and a mindful approach to eating. This comprehensive understanding and approach to weight not only aid in achieving a healthy body weight but also promote overall well-being and long-term health.

Regular Exercise: A Key Component

Regular exercise is a fundamental aspect of a healthy lifestyle. Its benefits go far beyond burning calories; it's about strengthening and energizing the body, enhancing overall health, and improving quality of life. Engaging in regular physical activity is essential for maintaining muscle mass, boosting metabolism, and positively influencing body composition.

Exercise plays a crucial role in overall health and well-being. It strengthens the heart and improves circulation, which can reduce the risk of heart disease and stroke. Regular physical activity also enhances lung capacity and efficiency, boosts the immune system, and improves mental health by reducing symptoms of depression and anxiety. Furthermore, exercise helps in managing blood sugar and insulin levels, reducing the risk of type 2 diabetes.

Finding Enjoyable Activities

One of the keys to maintaining a regular exercise routine is finding activities that you enjoy. When exercise is enjoyable, it becomes something to look forward to rather than a chore, increasing the likelihood of sustaining it long-term.

Enjoyable activities vary from person to person. Some may find joy in solitary activities like walking, running, or swimming, while others may prefer group activities like dance classes, team sports, or cycling groups. The variety and versatility of exercise mean that there is an activity suited to every individual's preferences and lifestyle.

The Importance of Strength Training

Strength training, also known as resistance training, plays a vital role in maintaining muscle mass, which is important for a healthy metabolism. As we age, muscle mass naturally decreases, leading to a slower metabolism. Strength training can counteract this process, helping to maintain and build muscle mass.

In addition to boosting metabolism, strength training also improves body composition – the ratio of fat to muscle in the body. Increased muscle mass leads to a leaner physique and can improve overall health by reducing the risk of obesity-related diseases. It also enhances bone density, reducing the risk of osteoporosis, and improves balance and coordination.

The Psychology of Weight Management

Weight management extends far beyond the physical aspects of diet and exercise. It encompasses a significant psychological component that plays a crucial role in how individuals approach and maintain a healthy weight. Understanding and addressing these psychological aspects is essential for achieving long-term success in weight management.

Emotional Eating

Emotional eating is a common challenge in the journey of weight management. It involves eating in response to feelings rather than hunger cues. The first step in addressing emotional eating is to recognize the patterns. This involves being aware of the triggers that lead to eating when not physically hungry, such as stress, boredom, sadness, or even joy.

Once these patterns are recognized, the next step is to find healthier ways to cope with these emotions. This might involve practices like mindfulness, which can help in recognizing emotional versus physical hunger, or engaging in activities that relieve stress without involving food.

For some, emotional eating can be a persistent challenge that might require professional support. Therapists or counselors can help in understanding the underlying causes of emotional eating and developing strategies to overcome it.

Body Positivity

Body positivity plays a significant role in weight management. It's about shifting focus from appearance to appreciating the body for its capabilities and strengths. A body-positive attitude encourages self-acceptance and respect for one's body, regardless of its size or shape. This approach helps in breaking the cycle of negative self-talk and unrealistic body standards that can hamper healthy weight management.

When individuals appreciate their bodies, they are more likely to engage in behaviors that honor and care for their bodies. This can lead to more sustainable and health-focused lifestyle choices, rather than choices driven by societal pressure or self-criticism. Body positivity also involves reducing the emphasis on the scale as a sole measure of health and success. It encourages a more holistic view of health that includes physical, emotional, and psychological well-being.

Overcoming Weight Loss Challenges

Weight loss and maintenance are journeys that often come with unique challenges and hurdles. Understanding and effectively managing these challenges is crucial for achieving and maintaining a healthy weight. Success in weight loss is not just about losing pounds but involves a comprehensive approach to changing lifestyle habits and addressing the underlying factors that contribute to weight gain.

Plateaus and Setbacks

It's common to experience plateaus and setbacks in the weight loss journey. A plateau is a period where, despite continued efforts, there is no significant change in weight. Setbacks, on the other hand, are moments when you might temporarily revert to old habits or gain back some weight. These experiences are normal and can be due to various reasons, including physiological changes in the body.

When encountering a plateau, it may be necessary to reassess and adapt your diet and exercise routine. Sometimes, the body gets used to a certain regime, and making changes can jumpstart progress again. It's also essential to look at other aspects of health, such as sleep and stress, which can impact weight loss.

Overcoming setbacks requires patience and perseverance. It's important to not let temporary slip-ups derail the overall goal. Refocusing on your objectives and understanding that progress is not always linear can help in getting back on track.

Sustainable Changes

For long-term success in weight management, it's more effective to make small, sustainable changes rather than resorting to drastic, short-term measures. Crash diets or extreme workout regimens might offer quick results, but they are often not sustainable in the long run and can even be harmful to health.

Incorporating gradual changes into your lifestyle, such as adding more fruits and vegetables to your diet, reducing portion sizes, and increasing physical activity in a way that fits your routine, is more likely to result in lasting weight loss. Sustainable changes also mean adopting habits that you can maintain in the long term without feeling deprived or overwhelmed.

The Impact of Lifestyle

Maintaining a healthy weight is influenced by various aspects of your lifestyle, not just diet and exercise. Factors such as sleep, stress management, and daily routines all play a significant role.

Sleep and Weight

The relationship between sleep and weight management is complex and significant. Adequate sleep is a critical component of a healthy weight management strategy. Sleep affects the body's regulation of hunger and appetite hormones, such as ghrelin and leptin. Ghrelin signals hunger to the brain, while leptin signals satiety. Poor sleep can disrupt the balance of these hormones, leading to increased hunger and appetite, making it more challenging to maintain or achieve a healthy weight.

Inadequate sleep can also affect the body's metabolism. It can slow down the metabolic rate, which can contribute to weight gain. To support weight management efforts, it is crucial to focus on getting adequate and quality sleep. This involves establishing a regular sleep schedule, creating a restful sleeping environment, and practicing good sleep hygiene, such as limiting screen time before bed and ensuring the bedroom is conducive to rest.

Stress and Weight

Stress plays a pivotal role in weight management. High levels of stress can lead to weight gain and make it challenging to lose weight. Stress often triggers emotional eating, where individuals turn to food for comfort, leading to overeating and weight gain. This type of eating is typically reactive and not based on physical hunger cues.

Chronic stress can also disrupt sleep patterns and daily routines, further complicating weight management efforts. Incorporating stress management techniques into daily life can help mitigate its impact on weight. Practices such as meditation, yoga, regular physical activity, or engaging in enjoyable hobbies can effectively reduce stress levels. These practices not only help in managing stress but also improve overall well-being, which can have a positive effect on weight management efforts.

Understanding the impact of lifestyle factors such as sleep and stress on weight management is crucial. By addressing these elements, individuals can develop a more holistic and effective approach to managing their weight. This involves not only focusing on diet and exercise but also ensuring adequate sleep and effective stress management. By doing so, individuals enhance their chances of success in achieving and maintaining a healthy weight, leading to improved overall health and well-being.

The Role of Community and Support

The journey to achieving and maintaining a healthy weight is often more successful and sustainable when supported by a community. Human beings are inherently social, and the encouragement, motivation, and accountability provided by others can be powerful tools in the pursuit of health goals. A supportive community can come in various forms, including family, friends, support groups, or online communities.

Finding Support

Finding the right kind of support is crucial in this journey. For many, this support may come from family members and friends who encourage healthy eating habits, join in exercise routines, or provide emotional support during challenging times. However, not everyone may have this kind of support readily available in their personal circles. In such cases, seeking external support becomes important.

Engaging with community groups or enrolling in weight management programs offers the opportunity to connect with others who share similar goals and challenges. These groups often provide a platform for sharing experiences, tips, and strategies for weight management, making the journey less isolating and more manageable. Online forums and social media groups can also offer a sense of community and are particularly useful for those who prefer digital interaction or have limited access to in-person groups.

The benefit of being part of a supportive community lies not just in receiving encouragement but also in the accountability it provides. Sharing goals and progress with others can increase the commitment to these goals. Additionally, being part of a community can lead to the discovery of new ideas and methods for weight management that one might not have considered before.

The Health Benefits of Maintaining a Healthy Weight

Maintaining a healthy weight is not just about physical appearance; it has profound health implications. A healthy weight reduces the risk of many chronic diseases, including type 2 diabetes, heart disease, stroke, and certain types of cancer. It also has a positive impact on the musculoskeletal system, reducing the risk of osteoarthritis and improving mobility.

Beyond these physical health benefits, maintaining a healthy weight also enhances overall quality of life. It can lead to higher energy levels, improved self-esteem, and a better mood. The psychological benefits are significant, as achieving and maintaining a healthy weight can lead to a sense of accomplishment and an improved body image.

In conclusion, the role of community and support in weight management cannot be understated. Engaging with supportive networks, whether they be in-person or online, provides encouragement, motivation, and accountability, all of which are crucial for success. Furthermore, the health benefits of maintaining a healthy weight extend far beyond physical well-being, positively impacting mental and emotional health and overall quality of life.

Conclusion

In conclusion, maintaining a healthy weight is about nurturing your body through a balanced diet, regular exercise, and a healthy lifestyle. It's a holistic approach that considers not just the physical aspects but also the psychological and emotional facets of health. Remember, the goal is not to chase an unrealistic ideal but to find a weight at which your body feels strong, energized, and healthy. It's about making choices that honor your body and contribute to your overall well-being. Embrace this journey with patience, compassion, and a focus on balance, and let it lead you to a healthier, happier life.

Chapter 10: Social Connections

The Fabric of Our Lives: The Importance of Social Bonds

In the complex tapestry of human health and well-being, social bonds hold a place of paramount importance. Often undervalued in the pursuit of physical health, strong social connections are, in fact, foundational to our overall health and happiness. This essential aspect of our lives deserves attention and nurturing, for its impact is profound and far-reaching.

Understanding the Impact of Social Connections

Human beings, by nature, are deeply social creatures, and our mental and emotional well-being is significantly influenced by our social connections. The relationships we form and maintain with family, friends, and within our broader community play a vital role in shaping our mental health, influencing our mood, and impacting our physical well-being.

The Psychological Benefits

The psychological benefits of strong social connections are extensive and profound. These relationships provide emotional support, instill a sense of belonging, and serve as a buffer against stress and adversity. They are essential for sharing experiences, expressing emotions, and gaining diverse perspectives. Engaging in meaningful social interactions triggers the release of oxytocin, known as the "feel-good" hormone, which enhances feelings of bonding, trust, and empathy, and reduces stress. This hormonal response plays a crucial role in strengthening our social bonds and improving our overall mental health.

Conversely, a lack of social connections or poor-quality relationships can lead to increased levels of cortisol, a stress hormone, negatively affecting mental and emotional health. Prolonged exposure to high cortisol levels can contribute to a range of health issues, including anxiety, depression, heart disease, weight gain, and problems with memory and concentration.

Individuals with strong social support systems are often more resilient when facing challenges, showing greater emotional stability and coping ability. This resilience contributes to better mental health outcomes, making the cultivation of social connections not just a source of companionship but a crucial component of mental health maintenance.

Physical Health Impacts

The impact of social connections extends beyond psychological benefits to tangible physical health advantages. Research has consistently shown that individuals with strong social ties tend to enjoy better physical health. They often have lower blood pressure, reduced risk of heart disease and diabetes, and even experience longer lifespans.

These health benefits are believed to stem, in part, from the stress-reducing effects of high-quality social interactions. Additionally, a supportive social network often encourages healthier lifestyle choices, such as regular exercise, eating a balanced diet, and following medical advice and treatment plans.

Therefore, investing in and nurturing social relationships is not only critical for mental and emotional well-being but also for physical health. These connections can lead to a reduction in the risk of chronic diseases, promote healthier lifestyle choices, and contribute to a longer, healthier life.

The role of social connections in our lives is multi-faceted, significantly impacting our mental, emotional, and physical health. Cultivating and maintaining these relationships is an essential part of a holistic approach to health and well-being. By prioritizing and nurturing our social bonds, we not only enhance our capacity for joy and fulfillment but also support our overall health and longevity.

Nurturing Family Relationships

Family relationships, whether by blood or choice, are foundational to our emotional and social well-being. They form the bedrock of our support system and profoundly impact our happiness and stability.

The unique dynamics of family bonds, characterized by shared history, unconditional love, and deep mutual understanding, offer unparalleled comfort and security. However, maintaining and nurturing these relationships requires dedicated effort and intentionality.

Active engagement is key to nurturing family bonds. This involves consistent efforts such as active listening, where each member feels heard and understood, expressing gratitude for each other, and being fully present in interactions. These actions help in strengthening the bonds, fostering a supportive, loving, and nurturing family environment. The benefits of such strong family relationships are manifold. They extend beyond individual members and create a positive, supportive network that resonates through the entire family structure.

Quality Time with Family

Spending quality time with family is crucial in reinforcing these bonds. Quality time is about more than just being together; it's about engaged and meaningful interaction. This could be through shared activities like meals, game nights, or simply conversations where each member feels valued and heard. These moments are not just about enjoyment but also about creating shared experiences and memories that form the fabric of family life.

Quality time also provides an opportunity to pass on values, traditions, and coping mechanisms. It's a chance for family members to learn from each other, grow together, and provide a framework for personal development and emotional support. In today's fast-paced world, making time for these interactions is vital for maintaining strong family relationships.

Overcoming Challenges

Family relationships are complex and can sometimes face strains and challenges. Navigating these complexities requires open and honest communication. This means expressing feelings and thoughts in a respectful and understanding manner and being open to listening to others' perspectives.

When conflicts arise, tackling them constructively and seeking compromises is essential for maintaining harmony. Holding onto grudges or misunderstandings can lead to resentment, damaging the family bond. In situations where family dynamics are particularly challenging or strained, seeking professional help, such as family therapy, can be beneficial. Such interventions can provide valuable tools and guidance for resolving conflicts, improving communication, and deepening familial connections.

Nurturing family relationships is a continual process that requires effort, patience, and understanding. The investment in these relationships brings immense rewards, offering emotional support, stability, and a sense of belonging. By prioritizing quality time, open communication, and constructive conflict resolution, family bonds can be strengthened, ensuring that they remain a source of joy and support throughout life.

The Value of Friendships

Friendships play an integral role in enriching our lives, providing a source of joy, companionship, and a sense of connectedness. These relationships go beyond mere social interactions; they are vital for emotional support, mental health, and overall well-being. Friends often become an extended family, offering a unique kind of love and support that is both chosen and cherished.

The benefits of friendships are multifaceted. Friends provide a social outlet, a chance to relax, have fun, and share experiences. They are a source of emotional support, offering empathy, understanding, and a shoulder to lean on during tough times. Friendships also introduce different perspectives, helping us to see situations in new ways and encouraging personal growth.

Friends can challenge us to be our best selves, offering honest feedback and motivation. They celebrate our successes and help us navigate through the sorrows of life. The psychological benefits of having close friendships are immense. Studies have shown that strong social connections can improve mental health, enhance feelings of self-worth, and even lead to longer life expectancy.

Cultivating New Friendships

Making new friends can open the door to new experiences, perspectives, and cultures, enriching life in numerous ways. Creating these new connections often involves stepping out of comfort zones. This could mean joining clubs, participating in social events, volunteering, or getting involved in community activities. Initiating conversations, showing genuine interest in others, and being open to different types of people can foster new friendships.

Building new friendships requires time, effort, and patience. It's about gradually getting to know someone, finding common interests, and nurturing that connection. The process of developing new friendships can not only expand your social circle but also contribute to personal growth and a broader understanding of the world.

Maintaining Long-term Friendships

Long-term friendships, while deeply rewarding, require consistent effort to maintain. Life changes such as career transitions, family responsibilities, or relocating can challenge these relationships. Despite these changes, maintaining regular communication is key to preserving these bonds. This could be through frequent check-ins, regular phone calls, or making plans to meet.

Supporting each other through life's ups and downs, celebrating achievements together, and respecting each other's life choices are crucial for sustaining these bonds. Long-term friendships offer a sense of continuity and stability in an ever-changing world. They not only enrich our lives with shared history and memories but also contribute significantly to our emotional and psychological well-being.

In conclusion, friendships, both new and long-standing, hold immense value in our lives. They enrich our experiences, provide emotional support, and contribute to our overall happiness and well-being. Cultivating and nurturing these relationships is an investment in our social and emotional health, paying dividends in the form of a richer, more fulfilling life.

The Role of Community

In the broader landscape of social relationships, the role of community stands out as a critical element in shaping our sense of identity, belonging, and purpose. Communities extend beyond the immediate circle of family and friends, offering a wider network based on shared interests, geographical proximity, cultural ties, or collective goals. The sense of being part of a community can have profound impacts on an individual's mental, emotional, and even physical well-being.

Communities serve several vital functions. They provide a sense of belonging, which is fundamental to human happiness and psychological health. Being part of a community means being part of something larger than oneself, which can offer a sense of security and shared identity. Communities also serve as a platform for mutual support, sharing of resources, and collective problem-solving, which can be particularly beneficial during times of personal or collective crises.

Moreover, communities can act as a catalyst for personal growth and social change. They offer opportunities for learning new skills, exchanging ideas, and engaging in meaningful activities. This can lead to increased self-esteem, a broader perspective on life, and a deeper understanding of the world.

Engaging with Your Community

Active engagement with one's community can greatly enhance the sense of connection and contribution. This can take many forms, such as participating in local events, volunteering for community-based projects, joining local clubs or organizations, or simply being an active and involved neighbor.

Such engagement not only strengthens the community as a whole but also brings personal benefits. It can lead to new friendships, a deeper sense of purpose, and a feeling of being valued and needed. Community involvement also offers opportunities for leisure, learning, and expanding one's social network beyond the usual confines.

Building Supportive Networks

Communities are a vital source of support networks. In times of need, be it a personal crisis or a broader issue affecting the community, these networks can provide invaluable assistance. The collective strength of a community manifests in diverse perspectives, shared resources, and mutual aid, offering both practical and emotional support.

These networks can also be a source of inspiration and empowerment. They demonstrate the power of collective action, showing how individuals can come together to create positive change. This sense of collective efficacy can boost individual well-being and foster a more resilient community.

The role of community in our lives is multifaceted and profoundly impactful. Engaging with and contributing to our communities enriches our lives, providing a sense of belonging, support, and purpose. The networks and relationships forged within these communities are invaluable, offering a foundation for personal growth, mutual aid, and collective well-being.

Communication: The Heart of Relationships

Effective communication stands as the cornerstone of all strong and healthy relationships, whether they are personal, professional, or social. It is much more than just the exchange of words; effective communication is about understanding, empathy, and the ability to express oneself authentically. In the realm of relationships, how we communicate often determines the depth and durability of our connections with others.

Effective communication in relationships involves several key components. Firstly, it's about clear and honest expression, where individuals feel free to express their thoughts, feelings, and needs without fear of judgment or misunderstanding. Secondly, it involves active listening, where attention is given not just to words but also to non-verbal cues like body language and tone of voice. This level of listening facilitates deeper understanding and empathy.

Effective communication also requires a willingness to understand another's perspective, even if it differs from one's own. This understanding fosters respect and trust, key pillars of any strong relationship. Moreover, communication is not just about solving problems or conveying information; it's also about sharing experiences, joys, and fears, which strengthens the emotional bond between individuals.

The Art of Listening

Listening is perhaps the most crucial skill in effective communication. Good listening goes beyond merely hearing words; it's about being fully present and engaged with the other person. It involves giving undivided attention, showing empathy, and striving to understand the speaker's perspective.

Good listening transforms relationships. It makes the speaker feel valued and understood, which fosters a deeper emotional connection. When people feel heard, they are more likely to open up and share more of themselves, leading to greater intimacy and trust in the relationship. Moreover, effective listening helps to avoid misunderstandings and conflicts, as it allows for a clearer grasp of the other person's viewpoint.

Expressing Needs and Boundaries

Expressing needs and setting healthy boundaries are vital for the sustainability of any relationship. Clearly articulating personal needs helps prevent resentment and misunderstandings. It allows individuals to care for themselves and their well-being within the context of a relationship.

Setting boundaries is equally important. Healthy boundaries create a sense of safety and respect in relationships. They help individuals communicate what is acceptable and what is not, ensuring that their rights and needs are respected. Clear boundaries also facilitate mutual respect and understanding, as each person understands and respects the limits of the other.

Effective communication is the lifeblood of healthy relationships. It involves active listening, empathetic understanding, clear expression of needs, and the setting of healthy boundaries. Mastering these aspects of communication not only strengthens relationships but also enhances overall well-being, as fulfilling relationships are a key component of a healthy and happy life.

The Digital Age and Social Connections

The advent of the digital age has significantly transformed the landscape of social connections. The rise of social media platforms and online communication tools has reshaped how we interact and maintain relationships. These digital platforms offer unprecedented opportunities to connect with others, regardless of geographical barriers. However, they also introduce unique challenges that can impact the quality and nature of our social interactions.

Digital platforms, particularly social media, have made it easier than ever to stay in touch with friends and family members, reconnect with old acquaintances, and even form new relationships online. They provide a space for sharing life updates, interests, and experiences, creating a sense of community and belonging.

However, the nature of these online interactions is often quite different from in-person connections. Digital communication can sometimes lack the depth, emotional nuances, and authenticity that face-to-face interactions provide. This difference can affect the quality of relationships and how we perceive our social networks.

Moreover, the digital age has introduced the phenomenon of constant connectivity, which can lead to an overload of information and social interaction. This constant engagement can be both mentally and emotionally taxing, and it can sometimes detract from the quality of real-life relationships.

Balancing Online and In-person Connections

Finding a balance between digital and in-person connections is crucial in today's world. While online platforms are excellent for maintaining relationships over long distances and offering convenience, they cannot fully replace the depth and richness of face-to-face interactions.

In-person connections involve direct communication, body language, and physical presence, all of which are essential components of building strong, meaningful relationships. Engaging in activities together, sharing experiences in real time, and the physical aspect of being present with someone – such as a hug or a pat on the back – are irreplaceable elements that foster deeper emotional connections.

Navigating the Pitfalls of Social Media

While social media can serve as a valuable tool for staying connected, it can also have negative implications if not used mindfully. One of the major pitfalls of social media is the tendency to compare oneself with others, which can lead to feelings of inadequacy, jealousy, and dissatisfaction. The curated and often idealized portrayal of life on social media platforms does not always represent reality, which can distort perceptions and expectations.

Furthermore, excessive use of social media can lead to isolation from real-life interactions and can impact mental health. It is important to use these platforms critically and mindfully, recognizing their limitations and potential impact on well-being.

Engaging in social media and digital communication requires a balanced approach. It involves recognizing the value these platforms offer in staying connected while also understanding their limitations and potential drawbacks. Prioritizing in-person interactions and using digital platforms as a supplement, rather than a replacement, for real-life connections can lead to healthier and more fulfilling relationships.

Navigating social connections in the digital age requires a mindful and balanced approach. Embracing the benefits of digital platforms, while also prioritizing and valuing in-person interactions, is key to maintaining healthy, meaningful, and fulfilling relationships. By doing so, we can harness the positive aspects of the digital age while mitigating its challenges, thereby enriching our social lives and overall well-being.

Overcoming Social Isolation

In our modern world, characterized by rapid technological advances and increasingly individualistic lifestyles, social isolation has become a significant issue. This isolation, a state where an individual may feel a lack of social connections or meaningful communication with others, can have profound negative impacts on both mental and physical health. Therefore, actively combating social isolation and fostering connections is essential for overall well-being.

Overcoming social isolation often requires proactive steps. This might include reaching out to family and friends, joining community groups, or participating in social activities that align with personal interests. The act of reaching out can sometimes feel daunting, especially after prolonged periods of isolation, but the benefits of re-establishing and fostering social connections are immense.

Engaging in community activities, such as volunteering, attending local events, or joining clubs can open up avenues to meet new people and develop friendships. These activities not only provide social interaction but also a sense of purpose and community involvement.

In the digital age, there are also opportunities to connect with others online through social media platforms, forums, or interest-based groups. While these should not replace face-to-face interactions, they can be a valuable tool for connecting with others, especially for those who have mobility issues or live in remote areas.

Recognizing and Addressing Loneliness

Loneliness is an increasingly common but often overlooked condition that profoundly impacts mental health and overall well-being. It is the subjective feeling of isolation or not having meaningful social connections, and it's important to recognize that loneliness can affect anyone, regardless of the number of social interactions they have. Tackling loneliness involves both recognizing its presence and actively seeking ways to address it.

It's crucial to understand that loneliness is subjective. It's not about how many friends or social interactions one has, but about how connected and supported one feels. Even individuals with a wide social circle can experience loneliness if their relationships lack depth and meaningful connection. Identifying feelings of loneliness can sometimes be challenging, as it often gets masked by busyness or social activities. Signs of loneliness can include feelings of emptiness, sadness, and a longing for genuine connection or understanding from others. Recognizing and acknowledging one's own feelings of loneliness is an important first step in addressing it. Accepting that one is experiencing loneliness is not a sign of weakness but rather an important self-awareness step.

One effective way to combat loneliness is to reconnect with old friends. Rekindling these relationships can reignite a sense of familiarity and shared history, which can be comforting and fulfilling.

Actively making an effort to meet new people can also help. This may involve joining clubs, groups, or activities where one can meet others with similar interests. Making new connections can open up opportunities for developing new friendships and expanding one's social circle.

Focusing on deepening a few close relationships can be more beneficial than having many acquaintances. Quality, in this case, is more important than quantity. Engaging in meaningful conversations, spending quality time together, and showing genuine interest in each other's lives can strengthen these bonds.

Participating in community activities or volunteer work can provide a sense of belonging and purpose, helping to alleviate feelings of loneliness. Being part of a community can foster a sense of connection and contribution, which is essential in combating loneliness.

Recognizing and addressing loneliness is a crucial aspect of maintaining mental health and well-being. By acknowledging feelings of loneliness and actively seeking to build and deepen social connections, individuals can combat the sense of isolation. This involves not just increasing the number of social interactions but also enhancing the quality of these relationships, leading to a more fulfilled and connected life.

The Role of Support Groups

For individuals facing specific challenges or life circumstances, such as dealing with a chronic illness, bereavement, or mental health issues, support groups can be incredibly beneficial. These groups provide a space where individuals can share experiences with others who understand and empathize with their situation, offering a sense of community and belonging.

Support groups facilitate the sharing of personal experiences, coping strategies, and provide emotional support. They can be a powerful antidote to the feelings of isolation and misunderstanding that often accompany challenging life situations.

In conclusion, actively working against social isolation is crucial for maintaining mental and physical health. This involves taking steps to engage with others, recognizing and addressing feelings of loneliness, and potentially participating in support groups. By fostering social connections and community involvement, individuals can combat loneliness, enrich their social lives, and enhance their overall well-being.

The Joy of Giving Back

In the pursuit of personal well-being, the joy and satisfaction derived from giving back to others often play a crucial role. Altruism, or selflessly contributing to the well-being of others, can be an immensely fulfilling aspect of life. This may involve acts of kindness, volunteering, or engaging in community service. The benefits of such altruistic behavior extend far beyond the immediate assistance provided to others; they also significantly enrich the giver's own life, emotionally and socially.

Altruism encompasses a range of behaviors from small acts of kindness, like helping a neighbor or offering a compliment, to more significant commitments, such as regular volunteer work or philanthropy. These actions, motivated by a genuine desire to benefit others, can have a profound impact on the giver's sense of self-worth and happiness.

One of the key aspects of altruism is its ability to connect us more deeply with others. Engaging in altruistic acts can break down barriers, fostering a sense of community and mutual understanding. This connection to others can be particularly powerful in counteracting feelings of isolation or disconnection.

The Rewards of Altruism

The rewards of altruism are numerous and significant, particularly in terms of mental health. Engaging in acts of kindness and volunteer work can provide a deep sense of purpose and satisfaction. Helping others can lead to what is often referred to as a "helper's high," a state of euphoria followed by a longer period of improved emotional well-being.

Additionally, altruism can contribute to the development of a more compassionate society. When individuals engage in altruistic behaviors, it often inspires others to do the same, creating a ripple effect of kindness and generosity.

Moreover, altruism has been linked to numerous health benefits. Regular volunteers often report better mental and physical health than those who do not volunteer. The social interaction involved in volunteer work can reduce the risk of depression and anxiety, while the physical activity involved in many types of volunteer work can improve physical health.

In conclusion, the joy of giving back through altruistic acts is a critical component of a healthy, fulfilling life. Not only does it benefit the recipients of these acts, but it also significantly enhances the giver's own mental and emotional well-being. By contributing to the welfare of others, we strengthen our connections with our community, derive a deep sense of satisfaction and purpose, and foster a more compassionate and caring society.

Conclusion

In conclusion, the importance of social connections in our lives cannot be understated. They are the threads that weave the fabric of our existence, providing support, joy, and meaning. This chapter has highlighted the significance of nurturing these relationships, understanding their impact on our health, and the various ways we can strengthen our bonds with family, friends, and the community.

Remember, nurturing social connections is an ongoing process, one that requires time, effort, and heart. By prioritizing these relationships, we not only enhance our own well-being but also contribute to a more connected, compassionate world. Embrace the power of connection and let it illuminate your path to a fulfilled and wholesome life.

Final Thoughts

We have journeyed through a holistic exploration of what it means to live a truly healthy and fulfilling life. This conclusion aims to synthesize the essence of each chapter, weaving together their collective wisdom into a cohesive tapestry of wellness.

At the heart of our exploration is the principle of balance, as reflected in a balanced diet – the cornerstone of physical health. Emphasizing the power of diverse, nutrient-rich foods, we've discovered that every morsel we consume can be a step towards vitality. This foundational pillar sets the stage for the nine subsequent elements of a wholesome life.

Physical activity, as addressed in our second chapter, is not just a means to an end but a celebration of what our bodies can do. Regular exercise emerges as a key player in not only shaping our physique but also in enhancing our mood and protecting us against chronic diseases. It's a form of self-respect, a commitment to honoring our bodies through movement.

The third pillar, adequate sleep, is often underestimated yet crucial. It rejuvenates our body and mind, playing a critical role in every aspect of our health. The tranquility of restful nights goes beyond mere physical rest – it is an act of self-care that nourishes us deeply.

Hydration, the elixir of life, is more than a mere necessity – it's a vital source of energy and health. As we've learned, every cell in our body relies on water, making proper hydration a key to sustaining our vitality.

Managing stress, a challenge in our fast-paced world, is not just about coping but thriving. Through various techniques and mindful practices, we've seen how finding calm amidst chaos can transform our experience of life, making stress management not just a tool but a skill for a more peaceful existence.

Chapters six and seven shed light on the importance of avoiding detrimental habits like smoking and excessive alcohol consumption, and the value of regular health check-ups. These chapters remind us that the journey to health is not always linear but requires continuous commitment and proactive choices.

Mental health, a topic of immense importance, stands as a testament to the fact that our psychological well-being is as vital as our physical health. It's a call to be as attentive to our mental and emotional needs as we are to our physical ailments.

The penultimate chapter brings to focus the importance of maintaining a healthy weight, a harmony of mind, body, and lifestyle choices. It's about creating a sustainable balance that celebrates our bodies and nurtures our overall well-being.

Finally, the power of social connections – the fabric that holds our lives together – emphasizes the profound impact of our relationships on our health. These bonds, whether with family, friends, or the community, are not just supportive structures but integral to our sense of joy and belonging.

The Art of Wholesome Living is not just a guide to health – it's a manifesto for a life lived in harmony with our bodies and minds. It's a call to embrace each day with intention, to make choices that resonate with our deepest needs, and to find joy in the journey towards a more vibrant, balanced, and fulfilling life. As we close this book, let us carry forward the lessons learned, weaving them into the fabric of our daily lives, and transforming our existence into an art form – an art of wholesome living.